COURAGEOUS AGING

Praises for
COURAGEOUS AGING

Ken Druck is a national treasure! A magnificent man with a huge heart and a deep well of wisdom to match—he has never retreated from engaging directly—and honestly—with life's most challenging issues. In this wonderful new book, Ken explores the fears, aversions, and neuroses our culture has generated surrounding the process of aging. He joyfully debunks most of them, and offers us—instead—a clear path to reenvisioning our "elder years" as a time of great freedom, awakening, and vibrant living. He invites us to fearlessly immerse ourselves in the wisdom we have cultivated over the course of many, many decades. Our tendency to see the "senior" phase of life as a time of meaninglessness, irrelevance, and decline is unique to our modern western world. In *Courageous Aging*, Ken Druck assures us that the cultural paradigm we have bought into is not true ... and that we really might—literally— enjoy this sacred time more than all the previous phases of our life. This is a spectacular, ground-breaking book, and I HIGHLY recommend it!

—**JOHN E. WELSHONS**, author of *One Soul, One Love, One Heart* and *Awakening From Grief*

Other Books by Dr. Ken Druck

The Secrets Men Keep: Breaking the Silence Barrier
How to Talk to Your Kids
Healing Your Life After the Loss of a Loved One
The Real Rules of Life: Balancing Life's Terms with Your Own

COURAGEOUS
AGING
Your Best Years Ever
Reimagined

DR. KEN DRUCK

NEW YORK

NASHVILLE • MELBOURNE • VANCOUVER

COURAGEOUS AGING
Your Best Years Ever *Reimagined*

Published in New York, New York, by Morgan James Publishing. Morgan James is a trademark of Morgan James, LLC. www.MorganJamesPublishing.com

The Morgan James Speakers Group can bring authors to your live event. For more information or to book an event visit The Morgan James Speakers Group at www.TheMorganJamesSpeakersGroup.com.

ISBN 978-1-68350-448-1 paperback
ISBN 978-1-68350-449-8 eBook
Library of Congress Control Number: 2017901849

Cover Design by:
Rachel Lopez
www.r2cdesign.com

Interior Design by:
Bonnie Bushman
The Whole Caboodle Graphic Design

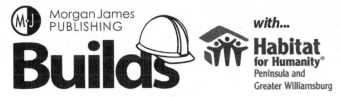

In an effort to support local communities, raise awareness and funds, Morgan James Publishing donates a percentage of all book sales for the life of each book to Habitat for Humanity Peninsula and Greater Williamsburg.

Get involved today! Visit
www.MorganJamesBuilds.com

To those on whose shoulders I stand,
and to those who will take courage
and inspiration from these words.

TABLE OF CONTENTS

ACKNOWLEDGEMENTS

I am a blessed man. And so very grateful. Being able to share what lives in me with you is an honor and a privilege I will never take for granted.

This work must begin with a few sacred and heartfelt thanks. I could not have completed this book without the love of my beloved mother, Roslyn Druck, who flew away this past year as her family serenaded her to "Somewhere Over the Rainbow"; my daughter, Stephanie, and her husband, Tony; my partner, Lisette, who stands with and beside me every day; my brilliant literary brother by another mother, Michael Levin; and my new family at Morgan James led by the visionary David Hancock.
KD

Introduction

AN INVITATION

Courage is the most important virtue. Without courage, you cannot practice any of the other virtues consistently.
—**Maya Angelou**

Getting older can be both glorious and treacherous, uplifting and frightening. Whether your hair is graying at forty, you're entering a midlife crossroads at fifty, running marathons at sixty, or blithely enjoying senior discounts at seventy-two, aging is no simple matter. Having turned sixty-seven this year, I have never felt so calm, confident, unrestrained, grateful, loving, or loved as I do right now. But I've also never felt so fragile, vulnerable, or—well—*old*.

So let's start by getting real. As we age, things can get better *and* worse. Take retirement, for example. Whether your career was out in the workforce or at home taking care of your children, the transition to retirement can be the start of a more relaxed, enjoyable life. As you look back on your life as a whole, you may feel a newfound sense of pride as you think about what you've accomplished. You may even feel overcome with gratitude as the door opens into this new chapter of life.

At the same time, letting go of your career may be painfully difficult. And if your job was raising children full-time, when they are grown and busy living the lives they have created apart from you, it can leave you feeling empty. You might feel like you're losing an enormous part of your identity. And that change might leave you feeling lost.

Two close friends of mine, Sarah and Jack, recently dealt with this exact issue. Sarah, a newly retired restaurant owner, told me how excited she is about finally having the time and energy to *really live*. Throttling back from the relentless stresses and pressures of running a business for thirty years, Sarah's feeling a freedom she's never experienced before.

"It's a new beginning!" she told me, smiling with what was practically childish delight. "I have my fears, sure, and my aches and pains like anyone else, but most of all I'm excited for what's to come. I'm a really happy camper!"

Jack also retired this year, and he's having the opposite experience. All he can think about is how "useless" and "disposable" he is. Jack feels like he's past his prime and is not sure what to do with his time. Dreading old age and fearing death, he's let his imagination take over. He's convinced that time is running out, and the best parts of his life are ending, or behind him. Jack's retirement has become a black hole.

So what makes one person feel despondent and useless while someone else, facing the very same circumstances, feels like life is just beginning? Even more importantly, how can we turn a time that many of us fear will be our worst years ever into some of our best?

Welcome to Courageous Aging.

Though we live in a society that worships youth and devalues aging, in this book we will unabashedly celebrate the great benefits of becoming our wiser, more seasoned, and very best selves at whatever age. Whether you're approaching midlife or well past it, this book will show you how.

You might be interested to know that Benjamin Franklin, a forefather of the United States and a renowned thinker, did not sign the Declaration of Independence until he was seventy years old. Or that Nelson Mandela, known as one of the greatest civil rights leaders in the world, spent almost twenty-eight years serving a life sentence in prison, and it wasn't until after he was liberated, at age seventy-one, that he became president of South Africa in the first election open to all races in the country's history. I could go on and on about men and women from every walk of life and every period of history whose enthusiasm, generosity, and creative juices were flowing mightily in the second half of their lives. Many of them have their best and most deeply meaningful years well after they turned fifty, not because they could still do cartwheels in their sixties and seventies, but because they were able to reimagine the future and *ripen* as human beings.

So the way that we approach aging has everything to do with the way we see ourselves and the changing landscapes of our lives. To test this, ask anyone over twenty-eight, "How old are you?" It will likely set off an emotional charge. We ascribe tremendous meaning and status to our age, often more than we admit. And we judge ourselves on a continuum from harsh self-rejection to boastful pride depending on how we're faring. We can move through the years and seasons of life harboring untold feelings of shame and embarrassment, comparing ourselves to the younger version of who we were, or to others. Or we can move through our years with enthusiasm and excitement, coming to terms with the past and dealing effectively with the changes that occur as we get older.

In these pages we will take inventory of where you stand on the issue of aging. Facing it all, from your fears and sorrows, including the fact of your own impermanence, and the possibility of losing people you love, to your hopes and dreams of finding joy, meaning, and peace. This journey will take curiosity, courage, and of course, *audacity*—the audacity to tackle issues you've been avoiding. We will audaciously come to view this new phase of life as a shining opportunity to reimagine the future and do what's necessary to have our best years ever.

Making that happen means embracing the greater possibilities for the second half of our lives and choosing a path of courage and curiosity over one of passive indifference and complacency. It also means rejecting dangerous anti-aging messages that, left unchecked, can become self-fulfilling prophesies. This will require that we put our houses in order. I don't mean your legal documents, though we will discuss that later on, both because it's important for the legacy you leave behind and because it can hang over you like a dark cloud. Even more significantly, though, when I say "putting your house in order," I'm talking primarily about matters of the heart.

Putting our houses in order starts with taking stock of our thoughts and feelings about getting older. It involves tending to sensitive matters in our relationships, those that bring our greatest joys, and our deepest sorrows. Putting our houses in order means sorting through and updating our goals and aspirations—because *yes*, each season of life affords us new opportunities for setting goals and living out our dreams, including those we might have given up on long ago. (We'll talk more about this in Chapter 9.) And putting our house in order means unveiling and paying close attention to what matters most in our heart of hearts.

At its core, *Courageous Aging* is devoted to helping you craft a vision for the life *you* want to lead and assisting you to step into that life. In the interest of doing this, I will continually invite you to reconsider every assumption you've ever made about aging and take steps to free yourself of the myths, misconceptions, and biases that stand directly in the way of your best possible future. Forward movement in the area of courageous living and aging, like everything else, requires your active participation and willingness to open up to a new way of thinking and embrace a new line of inquiry. By boldly entering the conversations "How do I really feel about getting older" and "What do I want my future to look like?" you are setting yourself up for success in addressing the tough issues and the hidden treasures of aging.

Much as we've been uncovering the injustices of racial and gender discrimination, it is time for us to awaken to the negative effects of age bias. Deeply woven into the fabric of our beliefs and attitudes about getting older, they can be subtle, pervasive, and difficult to weed out. Like racism and sexism, they are riddled with dangerous and misleading misconceptions. And they can be stubbornly resistant to change. Whether we use them against ourselves or others, age biases hurt and limit us.

It's time to set the record straight by calling out and clearing the slate of those judgments and prejudices we've been allowing to define who we are at fifty, sixty, seventy, eighty, or ninety. Being profiled, or profiling ourselves, as "too old" or putting these issues on hold stands directly in the way of determining for ourselves what our lives can be as we get older.

Now here's the part usually reserved for the "small print." Much of this will not be easy. Putting our houses in order—emotionally, spiritually, and in our closest relationships—will require willful diligence and some hard work on your part. Above all else, it will require a special kind of courage my older daughter, Jenna, called *strength of heart*. In this book you will be invited and inspired to summon your strength of heart as you get clearer and clearer about what really matters. For you, living and aging courageously could turn out to be any number of things, no matter what your age, including the following:

- showing yourself kindness, compassion, and patience as you face the changes and challenges of getting older
- facing and conquering what you most fear about aging
- allowing your heart to fill with gratitude, celebrating the blessings in your life, and then figuring out how to pay them forward
- opting out of society's blueprint for aging, which typically involves avoidance, denial, and youth-worshiping and, instead, fashioning one of your own
- taking the mantle of social responsibility as you consider what sort of world you want to leave behind
- making peace with *life's terms* as you learn to embrace the larger scheme of things
- developing an *honor code* for the second half of your life along with the health, spiritual, and interpersonal practices that make it possible

Why did my two newly retired friends find themselves in such different positions as they embarked on the same phase of life? Because each of us gets to decide how we interpret the circumstances that we face. One friend chose an interpretation that life was over, while the other saw great possibility for a new season of life. In the chapters ahead, we will free ourselves of the interpretations and narratives that hold us down and boldly explore the greater possibilities in front of us. This is the special sauce of courageous aging.

All of this magic begins with what I call the Courageous Aging Self-Audit.

"An *audit*?" you might be thinking. "But audits *stink and are something I avoid at all costs.*"

Don't worry. The Courageous Aging Self-Audit is like kicking the tires and looking under the hood of your car at 40,000 miles. Or searching your heart. It lets us know where we are now and which areas need attention as we prepare for our best possible future. Think about it: If life came with a "Fifty-Plus Owner's Manual," there might be chapters on "Reconciling Life's Terms" and "Processing How You Feel About Getting Older" and "Finding Joy After Fifty." But it doesn't. We have to figure it out and make it up as we go. Taking care of the real business of your life—so that you can live as fully as possible—begins with taking inventory. The coming chapters allow you to begin doing exactly that at your own pace.

Preface

HOW TO USE THIS BOOK

Have you ever had moments when you suddenly knew that you wanted to make some change in your life? For me, those moments tend to come at 4:00 a.m. Some weighty realization will hit me—perhaps along the lines of "I have to figure out what's next in my life!" or "I need to talk about this!"—and it's like a light has switched on and I can't fall back asleep. I *see* what I need to do. And I know it's time to begin doing it.

Afterwards, though, I face the more difficult questions:

Will I seize that moment of insight or just let it pass?
Will I allow an epiphany that could change my life to fade back into oblivion or live courageously and transform my life?

Will I resist these changes? Or will I persist by ushering in much-welcomed changes that I have pondered or delayed—perhaps for many years—and summon the will, and the strength of heart, to actually see them through?

To that positive end, this book comes in four parts. The first three chapters will help you take inventory of where you are, where you've been, and where you want to go next. By the end of Chapter 3 you will have completed your Courageous Aging Self-Audit and crafted a vision for your path forward.

Chapters 4 through 7 will then help you clear away your roadblocks—whether those roadblocks are regrets, denial, or losses—and move past any of the feared changes that go along with getting older. Whether that's the youth-worship that is so pervasive in our culture, or something else, we'll unpack it all.

Then we'll turn our focus to moving forward. In Chapters 8 through 11 we will do the work of putting our houses in order. That means taking care of our medical, legal, and financial future even when it also means finding new and audacious ways of turning our goals and wishes into realities. It also means navigating the complexity of our relationships with adult children and our own aging parents. And it means maintaining healthy relationships with our partners, even as we find ourselves changing in this new and different phase of life.

Finally, in Chapters 12 through 15, we'll shift gears. We will bravely face the fact of our own impermanence, and with that in mind, we will put what I call the *psycho-spiritual* parts of our house in order. We will express profound gratitude, offer apologies to those we've wronged as well as forgiveness to those who have mistreated us (including ourselves). We will rise to our responsibility to leave this world better than we found it. And, finally, we will make peace with what is.

But you don't have to read in this particular order to gain the most benefit. You can start anywhere, on any page. Every chapter describes some aspect of how we process our passage through this lifetime. And each section offers some degree of mastery for making these our best years ever.

Do participate as you read. You will find exercises throughout—and they're essential to the process of courageous aging. Participating actively as you read will help you own up to things that have been weighing on you for years, even as you're often unaware of them. To get you started, the Courageous Aging Self-Audit will uncover your core issues and concerns about getting older.

And yet this book is not specifically for those among us who are struggling with getting older. Rather, it's for anyone who wishes to make the good in their lives even better. For those who have gotten into the fruitful habit of continuously noticing and cherishing their blessings, who like staying a step or three ahead of the pain curve and who want to ascend to the next level of successful aging, this book is a perfect next step. It provides a structure for keying into the positive, while addressing the challenges, and then moving forward with intention.

You could call me the proof in the pudding. When I started writing this book, I knew I wanted it to be about bravely owning up to life's terms and living out this next season in the best way possible. This was the inquiry that was coming alive in me—and my incentive for writing. As my own life unfolded during this period, however, the book almost started writing itself.

In the middle of dropping down into the depths of these issues, my mother passed away and the nonprofit organization that I founded twenty years ago to honor my older daughter, Jenna, closed its doors. These changes cast everything in a new light. Although my mother had lived a long and full life, I was now faced with a time of grieving. Letting go of the person who had brought me into this world, been there in every season of my life, and nurtured me with her love at every turn, was more difficult than I had imagined. Letting go of the organization that had been the center of my universe and our community, as well as a lifeline to countless families for twenty years, left me facing my own fears about getting older. Both of these losses resulted in breaking new ground in the ways I viewed life, and in ways I could never have imagined.

During the same period, exciting new chapters of my life were also beginning. My daughter, Stefie, fell deeply in love with and married the man of her dreams. And that brought a whole new kind of happiness into my life. On top of that, I'm blessed to have Lisette—a woman I love and with whom I want to spend every waking moment. I've entered the most creative period of my life, which includes writing books, blogs, and editorials; doing some of my best coaching/consulting ever; creating a new platform for my speaking career; and getting involved in heart-centered community service. And finally, making my health more of a priority has left me feeling (and looking) 100 percent better.

I realized that my life had become a test case for this business of courageous living and aging. I faced an overwhelming mix of sorrow and joy, and it was incumbent upon me to find an honest and spirited path through it all. I found myself learning from experiences as well as from others around me, including the elders in my life, the brave folks in my Courageous Aging workshops, buddies in my "Goonies" men's group, and the dear friends and colleagues who helped me fine-tune the ideas in this book, hone my perspectives on aging, and inspire me to reach for the best in myself. The processes of writing and of growing older have shown me just how much we all have to gain by turning our age-related fears into newfound courage and clarity.

There's no cookie-cutter solution, of course, for becoming the best version of ourselves at this time or in any life stage. Yet it is incumbent upon us to do so. To quote one of my favorite poets, Mary Oliver, we travel this journey "without a map" and must call upon "the pioneer" within us and go by "the dim light of the stars."

So let's search together for that pale astral light to guide us, and in the meantime, know that your own vision for courageous aging will unfold on the pages of this book as you open your mind and heart.

TAKING
INVENTORY

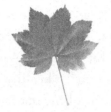

Chapter 1

YOU'RE NOT
A KID ANYMORE
(THANK GOODNESS!)

*He who is not every day conquering some fear has not learned
the secret of life.*
—Ralph Waldo Emerson

O ften it's an unexpected glimpse of our own reflection
that does it. Suddenly it hits you: "I'm getting *old*!"
You think, "Just look at me. I'm not the same person I
used to be. I've *aged*!" And if you've somehow managed to avoid
looking in the mirror, or in the light reflected off a shop window,
this can be a rude awakening.

Of course, it's not just your own image that gets you thinking
about the passage of time. At the Thanksgiving table you may
wonder, "How much longer can Mom do this?" or "What will
holidays like this be like after Dad is gone?" You may notice some
slippage in a dear friend's memory as they tell you something for

the third time over lunch. Or have to admit you're not as nimble as you once were, and rethink running 5Ks, playing tennis or climbing up a twelve-foot ladder to patch a leak in the roof.

It's true: You're not the person you were. But that's not bad news, quite the opposite. Yes, there are difficult and unpleasant dimensions to aging that all of us would elect to ignore if that were possible. Parts of this book examine those very areas—but in a way that's designed to support and empower you. That's because getting older also brings about a host of changes for the better—wonderfully positive changes. "Emotional freedom," "healthy detachment," and "spiritual awakening" are but a few of the many perks available to us as we get older. Yet our youth-obsessed culture either ignores, makes light of, or commercializes these gifts as it glorifies staying *forever young*.

Take, for instance, my friend Howard. At fifty-five, Howard jumped into a volleyball game at his company picnic and got outclassed by his thirty-year-old colleagues who were trying to take each other's heads off. Instead of feeling inadequate because he couldn't match up to the competition—as his younger self would have—Howard found himself laughing at the whole scene. Somewhere along the way, he had left his hyper-competitive, testosterone-driven identity behind and had settled into a more mature, confident, and happier version of himself.

A similar thing happened to my client Jodi. It came to her attention that two younger women at her company were fiercely competing with one another. Two decades ago, Jodi would have been jockeying among them. She would have been anxiously trying to carve her own fiefdom, believing success to be a zero-sum game in which someone else's victory translated into her loss. But no longer.

Jodi is now in her mid-fifties, and instead of competing with colleagues or ambitious youngsters, she mentors them. Helping them develop genuine confidence in themselves as professional women is a whole lot more meaningful than playing games and competing for her place as the alpha female. Now, when she gets home at the end of the day, she feels a great sense of satisfaction, rather than the fatigue of rivalry. The potential for more satisfying and gratifying relationships is very real as you get older. Another perk.

Or consider my partner, Lisette. As she and her friends navigate the realities of turning fifty—and are bombarded with ads for everything from wrinkle creams to lubricants—she carries with her a gem of truth that eludes many of her counterparts: confidence is the sexiest quality of all.

You probably guessed, from the title of this chapter, that I'm personally OK with the fact that I am no longer "young" in years. By the time I hit fifty, I had let go of many of the things that plagued me in my younger days. As a young author of thirty-five, I cared more than I'd like to admit about appearances, notoriety, and fame. My ego was tied up in gaining status/notoriety, power, approval, and adoration. And now? I may worry about those things momentarily, and then the *knowing* part of me kicks in. I smile and take a deep breath *knowing* I'm the best me that I can be. And that's enough. The confidence that I've grown in my mastery of the game of life, including the keen awareness of how little I really know for sure, brings a feeling of peace and freedom—yet another perk on the menu of possibilities I couldn't have imagined as a younger man.

It can be easy to lose sight of these deeper truths when we catch our reflection in the mirror or are faced with the passage of time in some other way and are hit with that sinking feeling.

When we're under the gun or experiencing a stressful time of life, we are most susceptible to old fears and insecurities. At times like these, the mirror can become our greatest enemy. One look at our older selves can send us back onto the well-worn path of fear, shame, self-deprecation, and other self-limiting habit patterns that we have never outgrown.

Many of us have internalized harsh self-criticisms that cause us to pass negative judgments on ourselves, highlighting what we perceive to be our flaws. Admonitions like "Look at those wrinkles. You look ugly!" or "You're losing your hair! You look terrible!" can play like broken records in our thoughts. And our conversations. And, all too easily, one look of disgust with ourselves can become the narrative for how we talk to, and treat, ourselves.

Sound familiar?

If you've been on a steady diet of self-criticism, or a binge criticizer who goes on an occasional rampage, it's time to change the conversation in your head to one of self-compassion. It may also be time to look into a different kind of mirror, one that reveals value-added changes in your heart and mind, rather than focusing on your appearance. Those of us who are used to being told, "You don't look a day over fifty," are blessed with a full head of hair, have a slender figure and wrinkle-free skin may be proud of our looks—even a tinge arrogant. It's easier for us to focus on the parts of us that are still "young." Whereas those less fortunate have to deal with the less forgiving signs of aging. And may be ashamed. Either way, learning to greet the older-looking, older-feeling version of yourself with kindness, acceptance, humility, and even affection is the key. Let's get started and find out exactly where you stand on the issues of getting older.

TAKING INVENTORY

I created the Courageous Aging Self-Audit to help you look at how you speak to yourself and to what extent you either deny or embrace the things that are changing in your life. You might have realized ten years ago that you were obsessed with seeking approval from others and needed some midcourse corrections— and have put that off until now. You may discover that you've already made significant changes in the time you take to "get ready" in the morning or before a night out because it's just not that important to look perfect anymore.

When we do a self-audit, it's because we're ready to take a closer look and hold ourselves accountable. Looking under the hood, so to speak, we might see a few things we can do better at. Or we might see how the experience of getting older is affecting us. We can acknowledge and appreciate ourselves in the areas we're doing well in, and find ways of being kinder and more supportive to ourselves in areas where we're struggling or see room for improvement.

Your willingness to uncover and face them all is as much an act of courage as it is curiosity. Do your best to step back and simply observe, rather than judge. And take heart. Every season of life has its daunting challenges. You know this because you've lived through them. This season, this moment, and this inquiry are all ripe with opportunities for newfound richness and meaning.

HAVING A LOOK UNDER THE HOOD

Great treasures are housed in the attics and basements of our interior lives. By the middle of life, most all of us have experienced unspeakable joy and gut-wrenching sorrow. My own life changed forever twenty years ago when a tragedy upended my family. My older daughter, Jenna, died in a bus accident while studying abroad at age 21. I'll share more about that in the pages to come. I mention it now because I know that in all likelihood, you, too, have endured circumstances that cracked your heart open, as well as ones that made your heart sing with joy. Due in large part to these experiences, you know more about yourself, and life itself, than your younger, less-resilient self could have dreamed.

Now is the time to unearth that treasure. Some of it will be uncomfortable, if not painful. Much of it will be energizing. Dusting off age-old dreams and fears, and discovering new ones that you haven't yet articulated, will give you the chance to decide—with eyes wide open—what this next phase of life will be. The self-audit is a powerful tool. It presents you with an opportunity to come clean about where you stand with being forty-eight, fifty-seven, sixty-three, seventy-six, or eighty-two and the opportunity to see where you can make midcourse adjustments. An honest look at our "inner lives," much like a review of our expenses and budget, requires great courage. The return on investment is that it frees us to imagine our best possible future, reset our trajectory, and take the first steps forward on a great adventure.

You take an educated risk when you do a self-audit. When you go seeking the truth, you sometimes discover that the truth is unsettling, or that it hurts. Your younger self might have passed on this kind of truth-seeking, preferring, instead, to look away. But you're not that younger, possibly conflict-avoidant or insecure self. Your wiser, more courageous self is seeking a deeper understanding—which is the reason you've picked up this book. The stronger, smarter version of you can handle a little discomfort knowing the benefits will be well worth it.

You may have selected a book on courageous living and courageous aging because you have a desire to become more confident, self-aware, and self-directed when it comes to the future. You may also want answers. At least some part of you is open to exploring whether you have allowed your fears, attitudes, and biases to limit your potential and to knowing exactly what they are. You're willing to face the critic in your head, and your fears, because you want to know what you're really dealing with. You have faith that such an honest reckoning promises a better, fuller future. And you know that the best, healthiest relationships, including the one you're having with yourself, are not possible without these kinds of reality/accountability checks.

It's also important to note that this is a *self*-audit. There's only one best authority on what's true for you and your life, and that's you. What you'll find in this book is a framework to help you discover what's true for you on your own journey of self-examination. In each chapter you'll find an invitation to be more honest with yourself than perhaps ever before. Becoming the best version of yourself in this new season of life demands that you go beyond the defenses you may have used to justify avoidance and inaction. In a way that's different from even five years ago, you now have the chance to live in accordance with what *you* want, rather than what anyone else is telling you to want. Doing a self-audit is the first step in this process of taking inventory so that you can discover ways of living even more authentically.

I can tell you this: It's worked for me. Though my PhD is in clinical psychology, most of what I have learned about life and overcoming the adversity in my path started with bold self-reflection. After the tragedy I alluded to earlier and transiting my own dark night of the soul, the falseness in my life began to fall away. Making the journey through (not around) adversity and fighting my way back into life taught me resilience—not the kind you can learn reading a book on positive thinking, but the kind that grows organically deep inside of you and leaves you humble.

Becoming a trusted resource and lifeline for families and communities after tragedies like 9/11, Newtown, and Columbine came from my willingness to face the adversity in my own life. I learned to embrace my brokenness rather than run away from it out of shame and embarrassment. Encouraged to "keep on keeping on" by family and close friends, I was able to summon the faith to go on. Learning to walk with a limp in my heart and accepting life's unwelcome changes without bitterness gave me newfound strength and hope.

Today, when I look in the mirror or a TV monitor at my aging self and have my own moment of unpleasant surprise, I call upon everything I've learned about overcoming adversity. In the loss of our younger selves, we're asked to summon our deepest resources for strength, faith, and courage. Transforming adversity is how we become the wiser, more authentic and resilient version of ourselves. As the late singer-songwriter Leonard Cohen so eloquently stated in his song *Anthem*,

Ring the bells that can still ring
Forget your perfect offering
There is a crack, a crack in everything
That's how the light gets in

It is out of our brokenness that we become whole. Out of the darkness, we find light. Out of our willingness to face into the tough issues of life comes the sense of peace, freedom, meaning, and connection we all seek.

You could liken reading this book and taking the Courageous Aging Self-Audit to purchasing life insurance. We don't buy life insurance in order to die. We buy it to live with peace of mind, knowing our loved ones will be taken care of if/when something happens to us. Now, as we contemplate the prospect of advancing years, we seek the peace of mind that comes from putting all the rooms of our houses in order. Rather than leaving our innermost challenges, fears, and dreams unexplored, we're going to face them head-on—and afterward, we'll enjoy the confidence of knowing there are no bogeymen left in the closet, no "I love you's" left unspoken and no important matters left undone. Feeling reassured that we have lovingly considered the needs of those we love, as well as our own, we're free to live the one life we have the best we can.

By allowing us to take inventory of where we are right now and to imagine some of the greater possibilities, the self-audit sets the table for creating our best possible future. Can you think of anything that tops living with peace of mind, a greater sense of freedom, and closer, more loving relationships? What other perks would you add? The self-audit is the first step, and then comes the new, improved version of your game plan for making these your best years ever. So let's begin.

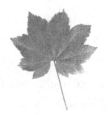

Chapter 2
YOUR COURAGEOUS
AGING SELF-AUDIT

There is a space between man's imagination and man's attainment that may only be traversed by his longing.
—Kahlil Gibran

The Courageous Aging Self-Audit is a process of finding out what's true for *you*. Everyone's path is different: different people feel different things, and each of us deals with our emotions differently. The same is true of our dreams. Our visions for what it means to have a fulfilling life are as unique as our fingerprints. The common thread is that it takes courage to step up and volunteer how you really feel about getting older and then step back and assess what you said, including the fears and grand visions you have never acknowledged. It starts with being honest with yourself. As you ease into that honesty, you may also want to confide in a trusted friend, partner, or coach, sharing both your fears as well as your excitement and enthusiasm for the new freedom you feel from leaving your old fears in the past.

At its core, this self-audit is designed to help you take stock of how you're doing with the process of getting older (at any age). Taking an honest look at yourself and examining the role age is playing in your life will free you to reimagine the coming years as some of your best ever. The road to creating your best positive future begins right here, right now.

Courageous Aging Self-Audit

Your Courageous Aging Self-Audit is broken up into three sections.

The first two sections provide a series of questions designed to uncover your innermost thoughts and feelings about getting older. The third section is designed to help you follow up on what you have discovered and to use what you have learned to create a better version of yourself.

Please take your time completing the audit, even if it takes a few days or weeks.

Like doing your taxes, you may want to resist filling out some of the hard parts. Instead of fudging or quitting, take a break and come back when you're ready. Completing this audit is a gift to yourself, as well as an investment in your own best possible future. Don't cheat yourself out of the discoveries that await you. Open your mind and heart to each question.

Section #1

Directions:

- Please put a check mark (✔) next to the age-related issues you might want to explore and better understand in the course of reading this book.

- Rate how big or small an issue each item is in your life, from 1 (small) to 10 (big).

- Feel free to jot down a short explanation of your response in the space provided, or on a separate document or sheet of paper.

1. The changes I notice in my body, skin, face, hair, etc.

① ② ③ ④ ⑤ ⑥ ⑦ ⑧ ⑨ ⑩

Small issue   Big issue

*Brief explanation:*_____

_____

2. Changes in my memory and ability to think

① ② ③ ④ ⑤ ⑥ ⑦ ⑧ ⑨ ⑩

Small issue   Big issue

Brief explanation: _____

_____

Section #1

3. Changes in my social life, and my relationships

① ② ③ ④ ⑤ ⑥ ⑦ ⑧ ⑨ ⑩
Small issue   Big issue

*Brief explanation:*_____

_____

4. My fears about getting older/old

① ② ③ ④ ⑤ ⑥ ⑦ ⑧ ⑨ ⑩
Small issue   Big issue

Brief explanation: _____

_____

5. My fears about dying

① ② ③ ④ ⑤ ⑥ ⑦ ⑧ ⑨ ⑩
Small issue   Big issue

Brief explanation: _____

_____

6. Changes in my personality that I don't like
(for example: "I'm not as patient as I used to be")

① ② ③ ④ ⑤ ⑥ ⑦ ⑧ ⑨ ⑩
Small issue   Big issue

Brief explanation: _____

_____

7. Changes in my personality that I like
(for example: I'm more patient and calm about things)

① ② ③ ④ ⑤ ⑥ ⑦ ⑧ ⑨ ⑩

Small issue   Big issue

Brief explanation: _____

_____

8. Changes in my sexuality and need for physical
   touch/intimacy

① ② ③ ④ ⑤ ⑥ ⑦ ⑧ ⑨ ⑩

Small issue   Big issue

Brief explanation: _____

_____

9. Changes in how I feel about life in general

① ② ③ ④ ⑤ ⑥ ⑦ ⑧ ⑨ ⑩

Small issue   Big issue

Brief explanation: _____

_____

10. Changes in how others, especially the members of my family and close friends, treat me

(1) (2) (3) (4) (5) (6) (7) (8) (9) (10)

Small issue   Big issue

Brief explanation: _____

_____

11. Changes in my ability to get things done (at work or around the house)

(1) (2) (3) (4) (5) (6) (7) (8) (9) (10)

Small issue   Big issue

Brief explanation: _____

12. Changes in my feelings about my closest relationships (my partner, children, parents or friends) (indicate specifically)

(1) (2) (3) (4) (5) (6) (7) (8) (9) (10)

Small issue   Big issue

Brief explanation: _____

_____

▬▬ Section #1 ▬▬▬▬▬▬▬▬▬

13. Changes in my faith and what I believe to be true

(1) (2) (3) (4) (5) (6) (7) (8) (9) (10)

Small issue   Big issue

Brief explanation: _____

_____

14. Changes in my ability to handle stress/stressful situations

(1) (2) (3) (4) (5) (6) (7) (8) (9) (10)

Small issue   Big issue

Brief explanation: _____

_____

15. How I feel about myself (and my self-worth) at this stage of my life

(1) (2) (3) (4) (5) (6) (7) (8) (9) (10)

Small issue   Big issue

Brief explanation: _____

_____

Section #2

Directions:

- Please answer each question using a blank page or a blank document on your computer.

- If you prefer to type or write in your answers, go to my web site, **www.kendruck.com**, and download a copy of the *Courageous Aging Self-Audit.*

1. Is something inspiring you to explore age-related issues at this time in your life? If so, please look at the boxes below and check the ones that best fit.

(1) A crisis in my life (circle the ones that apply): divorce, sickness, accident, change in job status, retirement, financial issues, or some other type of crisis.

(2) I just turned_____ (50, 60, 70, etc.)

(3) I've wanted to look at some of these issues for a while. This book presented me with the opportunity.

(4) Something else (please describe)

_____

_____

_____

_____

2. What, if anything, might be at risk if I maintain my current attitudes, feelings, and ideas about getting older? What benefits might there be?

3. What, if anything, might be at risk if I adopt a new, different, or better trajectory for the future? What benefits might there be?

4. A few things I'm dreading as I get older are:

_____

5. A few things I'm looking forward to as I get older are: _____

6. Are you at peace with, grateful to, appreciative of your younger self? If so, how?

7. Might you be grieving the loss of your younger self? If so, how?

8. Do you ever say or do things to appear younger? If so, how and when?

9. Have you experienced a time or situation when you suddenly felt "old?" Describe how and when this happened.

10. In what ways might you have avoided dealing with getting older?

█████████████████████████████████████ Section #2 ████████

11. Are there a few things you need to work on and improve when it comes to aging? If so, what are they?

12. When it comes to how you feel about getting older, what would be a good thing to change if you could?

13. When it comes to getting older, what guiding principles have you adopted, or would be good for you to adopt?

14. What weighs most heavily on your heart as you think about getting older?

15. What parts of your legal and financial life still need to be handled so your loved ones are taken care of should you die or become disabled?

16. Please describe your ideal life as you get older, in the following areas:

- My Physical Health
- My Mental and Emotional Health and Well Being
- My Relationships/Family Life
- My Spirituality and Faith
- My Activity, i.e., Work Life/Job/Community Involvement
- My Play, Fun, Adventures, and Social Activities
- My Curiosities and Thirst for Lifelong Learning

17. How long do you expect to live? Is there anything you could do that might improve the quality and length of your life? If so, what is it?

18. Have you spoken to those you love about death and/or communicated your wishes should you die? If so, what have you told them? If not, do you plan on doing this and when? What will you want to tell them?

19. Please describe the ideal conditions under which you'd like to age. Be specific about where you're living, who is there, what you're doing, how you're feeling, etc.

20. Please describe the ideal conditions under which you'd like to die, when the time comes.

21. Please say in a few sentences what you would like your legacy to be and how you wish to be remembered.

Section #3
Exploring the Results of Your Self-Audit

1. First, congratulate yourself. You've just taken a brave and important step forward on the path of courageous living/aging.

2. Please go back and circle or highlight Hot Spots (i.e. the issues that are the most emotionally charged, disturbing or exciting, or that you'll want to revisit). Review your self-audit after reading this book to see if the issues that were identified as Hot Spots have shifted.

3. Write these highlighted issues down as "My Courageous Aging Work Agenda". Take each item on your list into your thoughts, meditations, moments of reflection/contemplation, prayer, exploration and/or private conversations.

4. To best ensure following through on and integrating what you've learned, consider sharing the results of your audit with a trusted confidant, be they a family member, close friend, counselor or coach. Sign up for a workshop/class/conference/support group or a courageous living discussion group in your community (see guidelines for starting a discussion group or a book club on my website www.kendruck.com). Look within and formulate your own plan for your best possible future.

DOING THE (INNER) WORK

It takes a whole lot of strength and humility to engage in this kind of deep reflection and do the inner work necessary to grow our souls. This type of bravery may be different from anything you've had to summon before. It certainly was for Susan, my client, after her life was turned upside down.

At fifty-five, Susan had spent a good fifteen years avoiding every possible uncomfortable feeling about getting older. She had employed a wide variety of delay and diversionary tactics including cosmetic surgery, Botox, expensive clothing and jewelry, and costly wrinkle creams. She was also a master of redirecting conversations away from issues of aging, and—when none of those interventions did the trick—she would self-medicate with prescription drugs and several glasses of white wine. In all those years, Susan had always managed to stay one step ahead of her fears. Or so she thought.

Then her best friend from childhood, Barb, was diagnosed with ALS. In a matter of months Barb lost nearly all her ability to move, including her ability to speak. Susan was right by her friend's side as Barb's loss of function worsened over the months. And then, with Susan, her husband, and her children at her bedside, Barb quietly passed away.

Barb's death was the worst thing Susan had ever faced. She was inescapably devastated. Suddenly none of her usual escape tactics worked. For the first time in her life, she had no way of dealing with her fear and sorrow.

"I've been running away from this kind of thing my whole life," she told me at our first coaching session. "I'm tired of running but I have no idea what else there is," she confessed.

It's safe to say that Susan had effectively skipped "Coping with Adversity 101." She had never allowed herself to face challenging circumstances in an honest way, and she had never looked under the hood to see what was driving her.

Barb's illness was an awakening. Susan had summoned the courage to remain by her friend's side through the entire ordeal. That meant that she had now looked directly at illness, decline, and death—and allowed herself to feel the intense sorrow, an emotion she had long denied. For Susan, dealing with her best friend's illness and passing was a powerful entrée into her own fears about getting older. At last she was ready to look unflinchingly at herself and the fears from which she'd been running.

Several months into our coaching, Susan agreed to do the Courageous Aging Audit. It took her a while to answer all the questions and she later confessed that, at one point, she was close to throwing it in the garbage. After all, Susan had spent so much time, and invested so much of herself, in hiding, denying, repressing, and avoiding her discomfort around getting/being older.

"Barb was always on me about this," Susan told me, as she handed me her completed audit. "She would want me to be brutally honest and I was." Sure enough, Susan had downloaded the full measure of her fears about aging, which included a stockpile of disdain, self-loathing, and feelings of worthlessness—all of which became the focus of our coaching sessions.

After a few months of retraining herself to move *toward* her uncomfortable feelings rather than away from them, it started to feel a little more natural to her. Then she began to experience a sense of relief. It was very different from the relief she'd drawn from alcohol, spa treatments, and cosmetic surgery. Susan had been holding so tightly to a younger "more attractive and therefore lovable" version of herself; now she began to investigate the fear of getting old beneath that tight grasp.

As we talked, what surfaced was a sense of despair that was even more debilitating than her fear—that of having never really lived. Not only had Susan barricaded herself behind wall of fear, shame, and self-loathing, she had allowed these things to stand in the way of finding her joy. There were so many things she still wanted to do. But she was too afraid to dream them, much less do them. Grieving the things that her best friend, Barb, would never get to experience was a doorway to discovering her own dreams and innermost desires.

Susan found herself embarking on a whole new way of being even as she grieved. Having excavated some of her old passions—and some things as simple as hobbies that she used to love but had abandoned for one reason or another—she began to rearrange her priorities. "I am becoming a new version of me," she told me as she let go of old fears to which she'd been clinging so tightly. Susan started to feel comfortable in her own skin in a way that she never had before. It translated into a radiating confidence. A softening of her heart. And a smile.

"I like to imagine Barb telling me how proud she is," she told me tearfully.

Susan had invested so much of herself in always moving forward and keeping up appearances. Indeed, many of us have spent our lives invested in our careers, in raising children, in juggling competing priorities—and none of that required the kind of bravery that we now need. But Susan will tell you: if she was able to do it—after a lifetime fleeing her fears—then you definitely can, too.

It's in our DNA to be resilient. We have the wherewithal to rise up out of the ashes of the past in order to name our fears, grieve our losses, let go of past resentments, and boldly face the challenges of growing older. This is the recipe for Courageous

Aging and an invitation to write a new story—one that harvests the fruits of past labors, revitalizes your relationships with the people you love, renews your sense of purpose, provides newfound courage, and affords you the sage wisdom, peace, and freedom that await.

With these goals in mind, we turn now to Chapter 3, where you'll begin to construct a robust, inspired Master Plan for courageous living and aging.

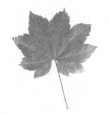

THE MYTH OF GRACEFUL AGING: RESETTING EXPECTATIONS

Your task is not to seek for love, but merely to seek and find all the barriers within yourself that you have built against it.
—Rumi

E xpectations are 90 percent of everything," a wise professor named Hallock Hoffman told me in graduate school. And he was right. When it comes to courageous aging, there's nothing more important to aging courageously than resetting your expectations about what's ahead for the future you. Too often, this means shifting away from a diet of fear, dread, and avoidance to one of open-mindedness, humility, curiosity, and courage.

James and Lora, a couple in their mid-sixties, recently attended one of my Courageous Aging workshops. They made their way through a minefield of issues related to their expectations about getting older—and how these issues were adversely affecting their marriage. When couples attend experiential workshops like this together, the benefits can be limitless. Not only do they get to see a side of their partner they may never have seen so clearly, or felt so compassionately about, they can provide a helpful reality check for one another.

Recently retired, James was quietly exhausted from his working years. His daily routine after work had involved a "decompression martini" before dinner, an evening of switching between *CSI* and CNN and, on occasion, participating in what Oprah referred to as "The American Mating Ritual" the first time I was on her show. After his retirement, James was lost and floundering in a world he knew nothing about. Lora was in a very different place. Doing part-time accounting work on her own schedule, and with the kids now grown and settled in their lives, she was ready to start living. Having spent years daydreaming about having the freedom to travel, she wanted to try everything from road trips around the US to cruises to adventure travel to helping disadvantaged kids and families in different parts of the world. "Just get me into one of those overwater bungalow huts in Tahiti before I die," she told the other workshop participants half-jokingly as James looked on.

Lora was heartsick that she and James seemed to be in such different places in their lives. In a brave move, she decided to put her fear, sadness, and disappointment on the table during a group exercise at the workshop, and braced for James's reaction.

To her delight, James didn't respond with anger or by getting defensive after she told him how she felt. At first he seemed just to be listening, processing what Lora had said. Then he spoke, "I'm kind of out of my league when it comes to this kind of stuff. I'm sixty-seven years old and just now realizing how much I love my wife and want these to be our best years. I'm just not sure how it all works."

Touched by their willingness to be so loving and open, I asked James and Lora to do something on the spot that I usually ask coaching clients in private session: "Please finish the following sentence for me. 'In my perfect world, we will _____ in the years ahead.' "

Lora went first, describing her vision. She and James were finally free to explore the world—together. For the first time in many years, her heart felt light and free. Rediscovering her love for James, and his for her, made her very happy.

At first very slowly, James then began sharing his own vision.

It was easy to imagine that this conversation was going to reveal that they were in even more different places than they'd realized—but that's not what happened. Lora's open admission of her heartsickness and mention of Tahiti was the start of something wonderful.

Buried beneath the layers and years of fatigue that were making James feel heavy and lethargic, he, too, had dreams. He was ready for a change but hadn't really figured out what to do with his new life "in a perfect world." The more he talked, and with a little help from me drawing him out, the clearer it became that there was a lot of overlap between their two visions. Lora and James, it turned out, had both always wanted to go on a cruise to Alaska. And they both loved the idea of devoting a week or two a year to helping kids/families in need. In a matter of minutes, color seemed to come back into James's face. Not only did he look years younger, he took Lora's hand in a gesture of reassurance that things were going to be OK. Drilling down into the details of what they could begin doing together, James and Lora grew more and more enthusiastic and hopeful about their future. And so did the other workshop participants who commented, "They look like they're on their honeymoon." By the end of the day, Lora and

James had awakened their dreams, dropped their despair, changed their trajectory and begun to complete a vibrant new Action Plan: Lora was on Vacations-To-Go making arrangements for a cruise to Tahiti, and James had already scheduled a coaching session with me to work through "the lost feeling."

James and Lora are a great example of what happens when individuals and couples summon the courage to open up about their reality—and are willing to trade in old, self-limiting myths and expectations, set a new course for the years ahead and draft a new Action Plan. Facing into and working through the tough stuff led them to a brighter now and better future.

It's time to ask you to finish the same liberating sentence about your own future. "In my perfect world . . ." This might be a perfect time to get out your notebook, open your computer file on Courageous Living/Aging and get to work answering that question with bold honesty. And when you're ready, let's begin to map out a vibrant Action Plan for your best possible future.

CRAFTING YOUR ACTION PLAN

The core of any successful, sustainable Action Plan is a vision for what's possible. By putting yourself on the line and stating your innermost hopes and dreams, you are creating a wonderful opportunity for mapping out the first steps of your new journey.

Generally, because we live in an era of anti-aging where how you look (appearance) is half the battle, "vision" plans are often no more complex than a picture of our ideal physique stuck to the refrigerator, in an effort to deter snacking. Of course that picture quickly gets hidden under grocery lists and bills, and the vision slips away.

And it might be easy for us to conjure up a vision for one single aspect of our lives: the fact that we want to lose ten pounds, how much more money we'd like to have in savings, which countries we'd like to visit, or where we'd like to live. These are slices of life, but what about the whole picture? How do we put *the whole picture* on the refrigerator: the vision for what we want to do with our precious time on earth? The purpose of the Action Plan is to capture that whole picture, explain why it means so much to you, and create a road map for how you're going to get there.

If that sounds ambitious, it is. It's also entirely feasible, as we have seen. You're now at a point in your life where you have a great deal of wisdom and experience to draw on. It might have been difficult at thirty-five or forty years of age to articulate a vision for your life and legacy. But now, when it comes to spelling out your ideal life, and even your legacy, the answers are right there within you. (You might have your doubts about that, but trust me—you do have those answers in you.)

Like the "In my perfect world . . ." exercise, there are many ways to free up your imagination in search of *the answers within*. If you're someone who has invested time doing visualization exercises, meditating, practicing mindfulness, listening to self-help tapes, talking with a friend or working with a coach in the past, you might already know what works best for you. For some people, letting their minds wander on a walk in nature, flipping through travel magazines to begin conjuring positive images, doing some form of expressive arts, or just sitting quietly and listening to soothing music opens them to untapped wisdom and clarity. If you have a method that works for you, please feel free to use it, and begin now to visualize the future you want for yourself and those you love.

Whether you have engaged in any of these types of visioning or not, here's a safe and simple exercise to tap your inner knowing. First, we'll go back to a time in the past to see what we can find.

And then we will go forward to glimpse your positive image of the future. Since not everybody finds visualizing useful, please also feel free to skip forward to the next page.

REIMAGINING YOUR DESIRED FUTURE:
AN EXERCISE IN TIME TRAVEL

Situate yourself in a comfortable and quiet place, and have a pad of paper and pen handy. You're about to engage your brain in a type of thinking that's very different from our usual tasks; it's not like trying to solve a crossword puzzle or searching to remember the name of a movie. Instead, it's about tapping into the far reaches of your imagination and harvesting the glimpses of happiness and peace that you find there into a vision for your Action Plan.

Let's go on a brief journey through time. Start by recalling what it was like to be ten years old. Maybe you're riding a bicycle or playing with your best friend or watching TV together with your family. Try to recall some specific details: the people, colors, sounds, the smell of your favorite cookie. When you have a clear image of yourself at ten years old, move on to fifteen years old, and then to twenty, but as you do so, focus on one constant: For each age, call to mind a memory in which you're smiling and calm inside. For me personally, it was a three-day canoe trip on the lakes of Maine at age twelve. Take your time here. Allow yourself to conjure up an image of yourself feeling happy about someone, or something, and being at peace.

As you pass through these memories of yourself at different ages, notice what's going on around you. Maybe you're on a boat dock watching the sunset with your little sister or visiting your favorite grandparent. Then take time to consider what made you happy in each of these scenes. Gently inquire, "What is it about these moments/memories that made them significant? What are the common threads that link these memories to one another?"

Hopefully, this brief time travel exercise afforded you pleasant memories from your past. Things that created happiness and peace back then may or may not afford you those emotions now or in the future. To see what happiness might look like in the days to come, picture yourself smiling in five, ten, fifteen, and even twenty years from now. Ask:

What is the source of my happiness and peace?

What's happening around me as I imagine this wonderful future?

What new adventures have I embarked upon?

What is making my heart sing and soar?

What is my calling?

What prayers are being answered?

Who's in the picture with me?

What are the sights, sounds, and smells around me?

Imagine as many details as possible so that it feels completely real to you. These are important clues. And this is a glimpse of the best possible future that awaits you.

Gently bring yourself back to the present. When you're ready, jot down notes to reflect the future you just envisioned. Capture as many details as you can to record the fullest possible picture.

• • • • •

If you did this exercise, here are some statements to complete that might help you clarify your vision:

1. **What made me feel good about my future was envisioning ____ .**
2. **What allowed me to feel this way was ____ .**
3. **What brought me peace and calm was seeing ____ .**
4. **What brought me joy was imagining myself ____ .**

These completed statements and the questions you addressed in your self-audit provide most everything you need to begin creating a blueprint for you best possible future. By opening your mind and heart this way, you're not only getting in touch with what makes your heart sing, you're forming the intention to make it happen. Add to this a keen awareness of the strengths you bring to the table, what most excites you, and what areas of your life are already in good order. Once again allow yourself some quiet time and space to answer the following questions, starting with your assets:

1. **What strengths do I bring to getting older?**
2. **What opportunities most excite me?**
3. **Which parts of my life are already in good order?**

Now that you've listed some of the assets you bring to a new Action Plan, be sure to include those areas that offer the greatest opportunities for improvements. These include the hot spots you circled or highlighted in your self-audit as your biggest challenges, the most difficult parts of aging and things you had avoided and/ or denied. These might be seen in our shame-based society as weaknesses, flaws, and failings, but in the judgment-free zone of courageous aging, *they all represent opportunities.* By reaching out to and supporting the young, unexamined parts of our aging selves with kindness, patience, understanding, and support—and sometimes tough love—we grow and flourish.

It may be difficult or even painful to answer these questions and delve into the ageless parts of our lives that we've denied and/ or neglected. That's in part because we're bumping up against the myths of graceful aging and deeply ingrained age biases that pervade our culture.

The myths of graceful aging are many. At the forefront is the twentieth- and twenty-first-century notion that medical science and technological advances will miraculously do away with all the uncomfortable aspects of growing older and dying. In 2008, a panel at the World Science Festival proclaimed "Ninety Is the New Fifty." But as a shrewd *Newsweek* writer pointed out, "No, it's not. It's not even the new seventy."

The aging process brings with it some difficult and unsavory challenges. This is an essential reality—and the age-related maladies that seem to come with getting older, like arthritis, can be as painful as they are unsettling. While scientists/genomics pioneers like J. Craig Venter of Human Longevity and Elizabeth Blackburn at the The Salk Institute are making great progress on slowing down the aging process, we are, after all, only human and mortal.

In the story you read at the start of this chapter, James had to acknowledge the fears and fatigue that were weighing on him so that he could clear the way for the future he really wanted with his wife. Addressing those issues head-on cleared the air and allowed him the freedom to begin discovering and planning for wonderful new chapters of life.

The differences between society's sad prescription for getting older and the life-affirming alternative, *Courageous Aging*, are profound. To buy into a myth like graceful aging is an invitation to deny the unpleasant realities of growing old. And try to make an end run around them. Thus denial and avoidance—not courage and grit—have become the hallmark of the aging process for so many of us. *Courageous* aging involves rejecting the rosy myth and acknowledging that this new season of life often brings along some difficult challenges. Learning to live with and even embrace these harsh realities is half the work of successful aging. Acknowledging that your physical abilities will eventually decline, and that you, like all humans, will one day face the prospect of your own death, requires more mental toughness than most of us have ever had to summon. You are also likely to experience the heartbreaking decline and loss of some of the people you love. And this can be devastating. It often takes every bit of strength we have to deal with these kinds of living losses and move forward.

Life contains some profound hardships. The good future is the healthy balance between the highs and the lows—because there are going to be both. Life is, after all, a package deal (unfair and more than fair). And all of this is written in the small print of life. The Action Plan you're in the process of creating will help you to reconcile and even transcend some of life's hardships as best you can, while cherishing what you value most.

Thanks to your review of the self-audit, you now have a fair assessment of where you stand with respect to getting older. Included in this is a summary of which elements of your life are most troublesome and problematic. And which ones are in pretty good order. And thanks to taking time to reflect, like the visioning exercise, you also have a snapshot of your best possible future. It's time to map out your trajectory. To begin mapping out how you will get from here to there, please jot down your answers to the following:

1. **Based on the results from my self-audit, the specific aspects of my life I most need to change, update, or eliminate (if feasible) to move forward are** _____.
2. **Some new things I'd like to add, expand, or explore in order to turn my vision into a reality are** _____.
3. **In one year from today the specific steps I have taken to achieve my vision are** _____.
4. **The steps I need to take this week to begin following through on my hard work and the promises I have made to myself are** _____.

With these answers, you've just completed the first draft of your Action Plan. In the future you will return to it and revise it, but what you have now is a powerful first step in the right direction. The next step is to put support in place to keep your forward momentum and hold you accountable.

In order to prevent your Action Plan from getting buried beneath grocery lists and bills, give yourself the gift of accountability. Share this plan with your partner, family member, friend, coach, trainer, sponsor, or perhaps even an assistant. Ask them for their support and spell out exactly what that involves. You might say, "Please tell me if/when I make self-deprecating jokes about my age," or "Please arrange to go over my master plan for Courageous Aging with me once a month to help me see where I'm progressing and where I need help," or "Please remind me that I'm beautiful just the way I am every few months," or "Please sit down with me and put together a fun, active schedule of travel, theatre, and concerts for the coming year." Enrolling support and spelling out what will help you fulfill your Master Plan will best ensure that it actually comes to fruition.

And of course, no matter how good the plans we make, no matter how detailed the visions we create for ourselves, or how much insurance we buy, life's unforeseen events will attempt to derail you. In the next chapter, we'll discuss the different kinds of unwelcome setbacks, losses, and changes that often appear in the latter years of life and resilient strategies for navigating the unexpected.

CLEARING
THE TABLE

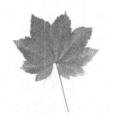

LOOKING BACK, CLEARING THE AIR: REGRETS, EXPECTATIONS, RESENTMENTS, GRUDGES, AND DEBTS COME DUE

Midlife is when the universe gently places her hands upon your shoulders, pulls you close, and whispers: It's time. All of this pretending and performing–these coping mechanisms that you've developed to protect yourself from feeling inadequate and getting hurt—has to go. . . . There are unexplored adventures ahead of you. . . . Courage and daring are coursing through you. . . . It's time to show up.

—Brené Brown

S ome of the hardships that life puts in our path make us feel as though we can't take even *one more step* forward.

There are times like this—stretches of time when most all of us have felt that way. Throughout my career, I've worked with grief-stricken individuals who have endured losses of every shade and variety. I myself walk with a limp in my heart since the passing of my oldest daughter, the family tragedy I alluded to earlier. This chapter takes an unflinching look at how, by honoring our wounds, setbacks, and failures, we can unburden ourselves of regrets, resentments, and grudges that stand in the way of actually having our best possible future.

A few years ago I got a call from someone I had never met, but whom I would soon know on a very personal level. I'll call him Jake.

Jake was a successful businessperson who had worked his way up the corporate ladder, eventually becoming CEO of a large company. He also had a wonderful wife and two children: a beautiful, active daughter and a son, three years younger, who passionately adored him. This little boy began following Jake around as soon as he started toddling, and he wanted to do everything his dad did. Jake began dreaming of taking his boy on the same camping trips that he and his own father had shared when he was growing up.

But just before the fall of what would have been their first camping trip, something seemed to be wrong with Jake's son. He was lethargic and weak, constantly batting colds and frequently laid up in bed. His once healthy, glowing boy was being pulled down by some undiagnosed illness.

Jake and his wife took him to see the family doctor, expecting a prescription for cold medicine or antibiotics. Instead, they learned that their son's condition was far more serious: hearing the word *leukemia*, their hearts sank into their stomachs and their lives as they knew them ended. They were told to begin treatment immediately and, "if it worked," their little boy would live "perhaps a couple more years."

"It's all we can do," the doctor told Jake and his wife. And he was right. Jake's son struggled through several years of invasive treatment and pain, and died quietly in the local children's hospital.

After several years of enduring the unspeakable ordeal of their son's decline and death, Jake's and his wife's lives were shattered. He had gone through setbacks before, of course, and problem-solving was in his nature; that was how he'd risen so swiftly to the top of his company. But this was foreign territory. The sorrow, pain, and anger seemed bottomless and unending.

A friend of Jake's suggested that he contact me. Reluctantly, he called and we arranged a meeting. He suggested that we meet at a Starbucks and I agreed.

When I walked in, I saw a man who had been dragged through hell and back. From Jake's appearance it was clear that he had gone many days without rest or relief from the emotional torment of losing a child. He was slumped over and could barely make eye contact as he told me the story of what had happened.

Jake described his feelings of hopelessness. Any future happiness would be impossible for him and his wife and daughter. He was certain that he would never recover and that life would never be the same. Finally, coming to the end of his story, Jake looked me in the eye for the first time.

"Just tell me one thing," he said. After a long pause, he added, "And please, don't give me any of that 'glass is half full' bullshit." I nodded, looked at him and assured him I'd be 100 percent honest with him. After a hard swallow, Jake looked straight into my eyes and said, "I'm screwed, right?"

I met his gaze, which was filled with the deepest despair and anger, paused, took a deep breath (to get over the shocking directness of his question) and answered him, "Yeah, you're screwed!"

With my answer, a weight seemed to lift from his shoulders. Jake was dealing with what most people consider the worst possible fate: the loss of a child. Yet just the act of acknowledging the truth—that no amount of spin could take away his inconsolable pain or undo the death of his son—came as a relief. There was no possible way to make it into something else. His son's life had ended tragically. And there was no time machine, rewind button or flux capacitor to reverse what had happened. No do-overs. No psychological or spiritual spin to explain away the pain and anguish. This was it!

Jake had sunk to the bottom of pain, drowning in the deepest sorrow. But by acknowledging (rather than trying to minimize or explain it away) the inescapable, choiceless pain he was in, Jake no longer felt alone. Or afraid. Telling him he was "screwed" (something I had never done before) was confirmation of something he knew at the deepest level to be true.

In the aftermath, his own life stretched before him, empty and meaningless. Not only had Jake's son died, his own life as he knew it was also over. The same was true for his wife and surviving daughter. The future they had imagined as a family was lost irrevocably. And yet the sun continued to rise and set, the world kept turning, and he had to find a way to both survive and move his family forward.

In some ways our lives *are* chaos. As we make plans and try to stake some ground for ourselves, everything around us is continually shifting and changing. Some of these changes disrupt our rhythm, some of them come in the form of pleasant surprises, and others devastate us. But in all these cases, it helps to recognize the chaotic nature of life or, as Jake later said during one of our monthly Starbucks outings, "We don't get to play God. What happened to my boy sucks, Ken. It always will. But things are the way they are."

This kind of irreverent acceptance—that it's OK that it's not OK—and that, in one sense, we're all screwed, is an important part of courageous aging. Parts of getting older suck! Undeniably. And no matter how you cut it, dying is not something most of us look forward to. Courageous living and aging afford us an opportunity to make peace with the ways of life and embrace its mysteries.

If it seems strange that Jake felt *better* after he heard me say, "Yes—you're screwed!" consider this: Sometimes the greatest gift you can give yourself is to accept what can't be changed. This means compassionately embracing yourself in your state of helpless unknowingness and sorrow.

ADMITTING OUR BATTLE WOUNDS

Most of us have wounds that have not entirely healed. Maybe you've been carrying around feelings of resentment toward a family member from an argument that happened many years ago. Or maybe you and your spouse made financial decisions that you wish you hadn't. And perhaps when financial and family pressures grew too great, you gave up on your own dreams—to start your own business or to do something creative. The path to your best possible future is not one lined with unforgiven failures, transgressions, and betrayals, or unreconciled regrets, resentments, and grudges. It is the clearing in the road that's ahead, after you've done your best to reconcile the hurtful, disappointing, and devastating parts of the past.

Now is a time to acknowledge the parts of your heart that may not have healed. As I said earlier, I have made peace with the fact that I walk with a limp in my heart, not unlike combat soldiers, refugees, and cancer survivors whose lives are changed forever by what they experienced in war zones. Try as we might to reconcile the hurtful past with revenge, positive thinking, or spin, most of us still carry it around.

In all my years of working in the trenches with people who have suffered the worst losses, I have discovered the most lasting and powerful form of reconciliation and healing. It is called self-compassion—and it is as simple as placing your hand gently, lovingly, patiently, and forgivingly on your heart. Self-compassion is the antidote to the shame and embarrassment so many of us quietly carry around. And it is one of the only ways you can make peace with and spiritually reconcile what you've been through.

So, are you willing to try speaking to your own heart with kindness? Yes, that's right—*talk* to your heart in a gentle and compassionate way and see what happens. Begin by thinking about something that continues to be a source of great pain and anguish in your life. Say what happened and place your hand gently on your heart. Using the voice of understanding and compassion, acknowledge your pain: "I can see how deep this pain is and how it continues to hurt. I can't imagine feeling anything but defenseless in the face of such sorrow. I am so sorry things turned out this way and I am holding you close." Let yourself acknowledge what you're feeling rather than dismissing, minimizing, rationalizing it away—or telling yourself, "Enough! Snap out of it! It's over! Why can't you get past this?" and "You have no right to feel this way anymore."

We can't alter or undo the events of the past, of course. Instead, now is a time to accept what can't be changed and listen without judgment to your own feelings—of every shade—about what's happened and how it has affected you. This is not the time to compare yourself to someone who appears to have simply moved on from a similar circumstance. Self-criticism is salt in the wound. Once you have listened to your own heart speak without fear of being judged or admonished, you're ready to turn your focus to what you *can* control: how you're going to live from this moment forward.

MAKING PEACE WITH YOUR UNWELCOME PAST

Sometimes we stubbornly hold on to resentments, punishing ourselves and those around us because things didn't go the way we wanted them to. Unfortunately, that's a formula for unhappiness.

Consider instead the following strategies for making peace with yourself—and your painful past—and then making peace with others. Clearing, the process of releasing anger and resentment, has been part of spiritual practice since ancient times. Letting go of and managing anger, and the hurt beneath it, has also been the secret sauce of my coaching/consulting practice and workshops for over thirty-five years. Clearing anger and finding your way back to Joy after a devastating loss like Jake's, or a painful setback, is different for each of us. But the following guideposts I remember by using the acronym FACE can help:

- **F**ace Into
- **A**ccept
- **C**ompassion
- **E**xpress

These FACE steps might not sound revolutionary—but they are. First, you've got to begin facing into the hurt, anger, and resentment that you're holding on to—and that keep you stuck in the painful past. This takes great courage, patience, and humility. Meeting with my best friend, Van, from high school at

Wo Hop, our favorite hole-in-the-wall restaurant in Chinatown, after not seeing each other for twenty-five years was more living proof of the need for good friends with whom we can reconcile the painful past.

"Can you believe it, I'm sixty-seven years old?" Van began as we sat down in the same booth we'd spent so many late nights in so many years ago. "When the hell did that happen?" he said half-jokingly and scratching his head in disbelief. After serving in Vietnam, Van came home traumatized, his mind full of inescapably horrific images. He had spent a good part of his life running, hiding, avoiding, and trying to escape the realities of his time living (and surviving) in a war zone.

Catching up on the years he had spent struggling to stay afloat after Vietnam, and my life after the tragic death of my daughter, was a reality check for both of us. Reaching back into the past and facing what had happened in both of our lives straight on was also a healing. Having shared our journeys, holding nothing back, cleared the air. Our tears slowly turned to boisterous laughter as we recalled some of the simple joys we had also shared back in the day. Owning up to how young, foolish, and arrogant we had been over the years added even more levity. And a soft breeze of humility and affection and self-compassion passed over our booth. Van and I were facing into and going beyond the painful past. And embracing the totality of life.

Dealing with what life presents you, straight up, can be harsh. Being able to share our stories takes some of the bite out of that harshness and softens some of the rough edges. Making peace with the past also opens the door to lighter-heartedness, as it did with me and Van at Wo Hop that night.

Saying how you feel and what you need is the lifeblood of healthy relationships. And authenticity. Honest sharing strengthens the connection we have with others and the integrity we have with ourselves. Expressing what you're feeling, getting things off your chest rather than bottling them up goes a long way towards helping you clear the air and make room for the positive future.

In using these simple clearing tools, you're also making yourself more capable of handling future challenges and becoming more resilient. Even as life has dealt you plenty of wounds in the past, there will yet be more daunting challenges in the future. While there are some things you cannot prepare for, building the strength, capacity, and character to handle adversity in a healthy and effective manner is always a good idea.

Aging brings along some difficult and painful realities. Some of them are subtle and barely noticeable, such as the sense of loss we feel when becoming aware that things just aren't how they used to be—and neither are we. Or they can arrive as a variety of obvious challenges—physical, emotional, financial—that crop up in our path. The pain of losing a parent, sibling, or dear friend may be obvious, whereas the pain and anguish of losing our ability to drive, to physically hear what others are saying at the holiday dinner table, or to bear children due to a change of life might be less so.

As you encounter new challenges, consider the tools in this chapter to be an ongoing resource. Whenever possible, consider acknowledging gently to yourself that your heart is hurting and needs to speak. As appropriate, apologize, forgive, and communicate your needs in a direct, forthright manner. And then turn your focus to what you can control about your life as it continues to unfold. Clear the air of regrets, resentments, and grudges and train yourself to notice all that is good in each moment of each day.

Indeed, this is a time when things may be changing—from your career to your social life to your home life, your appearance, and beyond. Life is, after all, a series of transitions, or, as a friend used to joke, "I'm in between transitions at the moment." The next chapter is about learning to recalibrate your ego and identity amid these changes.

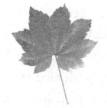

Chapter 5
FACING IN:
THE WONDERFUL WORLD
BEYOND DENIAL

If I have the belief that I can do it, I shall surely acquire the
capacity to do it even if I may not have it at the beginning.
—Gandhi

Sam's life seemed to be pretty much perfect. After graduating from Stanford, he spent twenty-five years moving up the ranks in Silicon Valley, always propelled by his charismatic, effervescent personality, technical know-how, and quick wit. Along the way, he married Erin, had two children, and eventually became the CEO of his company as it morphed into one of the most successful in the region. Sam seemed both indestructible and permanently successful.

Until last year, that is, when some big changes in technology and fierce competition from a rival company rendered Sam's employer, and his own position, "questionable." This new development came on the heels of Sam's purchase of a lavish home, both of his children's matriculation at Stanford, a steep drop in the value of his investment portfolio, and stirrings of empty-nest marital problems. You could call that a perfect storm.

For the first time in his life, Sam began to wither under the pressure. His fear started showing up in the form of panic attacks, about which he felt ashamed and embarrassed. It became clear to Sam that he was, for the first time in his adult life, defenseless against his own fears. Suddenly he couldn't ignore the fact that he'd spent decades on top of the world but unconsciously denied that his ceaseless drive to success was, in part, a cover for his fears. But the debt had now come due. Between the sinking feeling in his gut and free-falling into a state of panic every few days (including at work), he no longer recognized himself as the successful, confident CEO he had become. Instead, he felt like a waffling loser.

Not knowing where to turn, but knowing he could use help, Sam took a friend's suggestion and called me for executive coaching. And over the next six months, Sam went through a process of slowly, unevenly, and awkwardly facing his fears, one by one, recalibrating his identity, and meeting his "real self," as he called it.

It went slowly at first, largely due to the fact that Sam's go-to way of relating to himself when things were not going perfectly was with harsh self-criticism and scathing admonitions. He was continually demanding, "What's *wrong* with me?" and shaming/assaulting himself for being so weak and out of control. These kinds of cutting rebukes were constantly echoing inside his head—as is the case for so many of us—and he didn't know how to defend himself. So he pressed even harder.

Sam and I began with some simple yet powerful steps: Giving himself permission just to feel his fear and sadness was a huge step. At first the very idea of that seemed strange to him. But he took it and the floodgates opened. Sam's admission of his worst fears and the embarrassment he had been carrying around all these months helped clear the air. As Sam gradually began to convert his critical interior voice into one that spoke with a measure of compassion, the foot he had been keeping on his own throat lifted. In its place was a hand of support, patience, kindness, encouragement, trust, and faith. Finally, he could breathe and even smile again.

Things would not magically get better all at once, but after months of working on this internal shift, a very different Sam stepped forward. He had retooled himself at work and had come to accept the possibility that there might be some uncomfortable changes in his professional trajectory in the near future. He knew that his finances might not look the way he wanted. He was able to forgive himself for that—and, more importantly, for all the years he had spent secretly harboring his insecurities. He could now live in his own skin more comfortably than he ever had. And he could consider a variety of viable options.

These positive changes worked wonders in Sam's family life. He found himself wanting to repair and renew his relationship with his wife and open up more to his children. His "sinking feeling" and panic attacks became a distant memory. Knowing he'd taken ownership of his problems, gotten the help he needed and become a better, fuller version of himself put Sam in a position to turn the pages of his life, recalibrate his idea of success, and write new chapters.

AFTER EVERY TRANSITION AN ADJUSTMENT PERIOD

Sam's story isn't unusual. Sometimes our habits of denying emotions like fear or sorrow are so subtle as to go unnoticed.

Indeed, camouflage and denial can become a part of our persona. In a culture that sanctions and even reinforces avoidance by prescribing a pill for every pain, a fix for every problem, and a diversion for every moment of emptiness, it's easy for feelings that are outside our comfort zone to go unnoticed and undetected. That is, until life throws something in our path that changes everything.

As we're seeing, the challenges that come our way—especially in the second half of life—can be both eminently painful and full of opportunity. Sam was cruising along his successful path; it wasn't until things looked suddenly bleak that he started to examine himself and saw the ways he'd been blind to and harshly critical of some of his most basic emotions. Processing those emotions cleared the way for him to move forward in almost every area of his life—regardless of whether he could solve the financial and professional concerns that had precipitated his crisis.

For many of us, the process of aging itself acts as a powerful trigger. We live in a culture that reveres youth and—as we'll discuss in the next chapter—offers a whole industry of anti-aging products, services, and spin to camouflage, conceal, and outright deny the fact that we are getting older. Most of us buy into the anti-aging mindset at least a little bit, and sometimes we buy into it lock, stock, and barrel. There's nothing inherently wrong with using anti-aging products and services that make us look and feel better. They can be a perfect complement to the inner work we're doing on getting older. Coming to terms with the older version of ourselves from the inside out, dealing straight up with the realities, including the shame, embarrassment, and/or fears that arise with aging, lays the groundwork for reimagining our best possible future. Treating ourselves with respect and compassion and bravely coming to terms, rather than denying, the natural changes that are a part of life, helps us embrace that future.

Let's stop for a moment, go back, and take inventory. In your self-audit, which parts of being your current age make you most uncomfortable? Are there unsettling changes that you've been trying to hide, deny, or cover up? Answering these kinds of personal questions with brutal honesty can be uncomfortable. As best you can, try to simply tolerate that discomfort, because it may be a sign that you're getting close to the truth. And please remember to be kind to yourself during this exploration process; you're not going to change overnight, so be patient as you start to uncover some of the things you've buried or were not aware of—just as Sam did in a process that took half a year and continues to this day.

What's most important is that you face in and use the challenges in your path—whether in your financial life, the loss of someone dear to you, or the very facts of aging—as opportunities for taking a pulse of how things are going and using what you learn to make things better on all fronts.

The fact that you've embarked on this journey of courageous aging means that you don't want to shrink or even remain static in the face of life's challenges; you're actively seeking a more vital and meaningful path.

TUNING IN TO YOUR VISION

In Chapter 3 you crafted a vision for the life you want. In this chapter you'll focus on uncovering underlying patterns of denial in order to help you reach that vision.

As we have seen, one powerful way of doing this is through talking with a trusted confidant. Doing this in the context of your own, personal brainstorming session is a way to identify old patterns of denial and self-sabotage that could stand in the way of making your vision a reality. And then there are those random opportunities we all get with perfect strangers.

Consider Donna, a forty-eight-year-old woman I met in a daylong strategy session while serving on a community board. No matter what we were talking about, Donna seemed to have it all figured out. She was insistent to the point of pushiness during our strategy session. And she was unwilling to explore the options and alternatives introduced by other participants. During our lunch break, she told us that she was planning on retiring when she turned fifty, moving to Hawaii, and working part-time renting motorcycles and kayaks to tourists. She commented that she was "over men" and planned on remaining single.

Donna seemed conspicuously resistant to exploring anything other than what she'd already mapped out or dealing with/seeing things in any other way. During our day together, she met every comment and suggestion from others with a dismissive, "Yes, but . . ."

Usually, I don't reach out to people like this, unless they have come to me for coaching or consulting. But after lunch I took Donna aside and asked her whether there was something going on in her life that was causing her to be so hard-nosed.

This time Donna didn't get defensive. In fact, she admitted that she was just getting over the breakup of an eighteen-year marriage and having a very hard time of it. Donna shared that she had been feeling "old and ugly" since her breakup. What she hadn't realized was how hard she was being on herself. In the fifteen minutes we talked, Donna also began to see how the defenses she had used with her ex-husband and family since the divorce were spilling over into how she was acting with others. As we prepared to go back into our meeting, I told her how grateful

I was to have been trusted with this information. Donna thanked me and told me she felt "one hundred times better" getting all this off her chest.

When we regrouped after lunch, something about Donna was markedly different. She not only remained open as other participants thoughtfully discussed our community project, she teared up and told me she was reconsidering the possibility of having a companion sometime in the future. She even jokingly asked one of the other men if he had a brother. When the workshop ended, Donna left with a room full of new friends and the door wide open to her best possible future. She had not solved all the world's problems, or her own, but she was now aimed in the right direction.

As we've seen throughout the earlier chapters of this book, good, open-ended questions produce fertile inquiries. Answering questions opens new doors of self-awareness and possibility. As you cultivate your vision for getting older, here are some additional questions to consider as you break free of denial and face in:

- **What goals, milestones and markers, achievements and accomplishments, nuances and special blessings do you wish for yourself on the path ahead?**
- **What patterns or habits of denial are you beginning to realize you must address in order to become the better you?**
- **What small steps can you take in order to look at the reality of the situation and move yourself in the right direction?**
- **Who can support you in this brave venture as a trusted confidant? And how can you support yourself?**

Be your own best confidant. Listen to yourself, be tough when you need to and soft when that is what's necessary. And choose your confidants wisely! Surround yourself with people who help create better, more expansive options, not those who cause you to shy away from saying what you really want, or enable you to stay stuck. Conversations laced with subtle judgments, criticism and/or negativity shut us down, whereas "safe" conversations that are judgment-free enhanced by directness, empathy, good listening, and understanding allow us to discover the greater possibilities within.

Set an intention for yourself and put it into action. Life will continue to be full of challenges. Allow for changes and new life lessons that make your initial vision even clearer. Continue to discuss your plan with people who can draw out the best in you. Keeping an open mind will uncover opportunities you may not have considered. And finally, allow yourself the time to continually check in with your own inner desires—as they solidify, shift and/or change. The world of conscious wakefulness goes far beyond that of denial and avoidance. It requires great courage. We also need a keen awareness of how seductive and compelling the industry of aging can be and the resolve to create our own path.

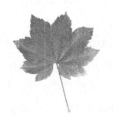

Chapter 6

THE INDUSTRY OF AGING: POP CULTURE, WRINKLE CREAM, AND ANNUITIES

When the only tool you have is a hammer, every solution looks like a nail.

—Abraham Maslow

The industry of aging—or I should say, anti-aging—raked in a whopping $260 billion in 2013, according to *MarketWatch*.[1] That dollar figure is a telling indicator of something much deeper that we can't precisely measure: our own discomforts, insecurities, and rejection of the natural process of getting older. Some of the products and services in this vast industry are genuinely geared to health, fitness, happiness, and longevity. These companies, founders, and employees are to be

---

1   Elizabeth O'Brien, "10 secrets of the anti-aging industry," MarketWatch, February 13, 2014, http://www.marketwatch.com/story/10-things-the-anti-aging-industry-wont-tell-you-2014-02-11?page=1.

commended for all that they bring to the table and how they are improving the quality of life for millions of people, but a great number of anti-aging products and services are designed to play to our fears and prey on our dread. They lack any proven value and can actually detract from the quality of our lives. This chapter is about navigating the sea of options in a way that helps you make good choices.

The distinct stories of two very different women illustrate the problem *and* possibilities for either disaster or liberation. For starters, consider that my sister, Roberta, would regularly see a woman at the gym who'd had an overwhelming amount of plastic surgery. Several other women had quietly commented to my sister that she "looked like Michael Jackson." And every time Roberta saw her, it seemed that she'd had a new procedure.

My sister felt sad for her and always made it a point to say a warm hello whenever they ran into each other. This woman seemed so desperate to look beautiful—and yet all the "work" she was getting was having the opposite effect. When Roberta told me about it, it nearly brought her to tears.

After not seeing this woman for several months, my sister was stunned to learn that she had ovarian cancer and had passed away. It plagued Roberta that this woman was struggling with a terrible form of self-rejection and had spent her last months pursuing cosmetic fixes.

Does the industry of aging prey upon women and girls whose fears, preoccupations, and even pathological obsessions with youthful beauty are out of control? Is brilliant marketing effective enough to convince women that a product, service, or procedure is the solution to one of the many natural signs we're getting older? Are we brainwashing millions of women and men into believing they will lose their appearance-dependent value, worth, status, and staying power unless they use a certain anti-aging product? And lastly, are we letting companies with millions of dollars of commercial interests hijack our mindset about how true self-worth is attained?

What had this woman in the gym missed out on as she chased a particular type of appearance that was beyond her reach? What does this tragedy, and so many others, teach us about learning to love and accept ourselves in the package we came in—and at the age we are? The better version of us and best possible future are not things we achieve with a complement of Botox or Viagra. They come from within.

The story of my sister's other friend, Susie, offers great contrast to this—though not necessarily in the way you might expect.

Susie was diagnosed with breast cancer when she was forty-seven, and she subsequently had a mastectomy. When it looked as though she was going to make a full recovery, Susie began to consider the possibility of breast augmentation surgery. Fearing she would be judged as disfigured—and unlovable—if she didn't opt for the surgery, she deliberated with her doctor, friends, and her family. And as it turned out, the most helpful conversation of all was one she had with her fifteen-year-old daughter late at night.

"Mom, you're so beautiful," her daughter told her. "Whatever you decide is okay. And you need to trust that it will also be okay with anybody you decide is worthy of being in your life."

Susie was struck by her daughter's wisdom. After their conversation, she kept returning to what her daughter had said. Finally, she decided simply to delay making a decision and focus on seeing herself as a whole person again, post-cancer and post-mastectomy. Rekindling her own notion of herself as beautiful—and as lovable—took time and great strength but Susie began to recover faith in herself. She no longer worried that she'd be viewed as disfigured or unlovable.

She also received the best possible news from her doctor: she was cancer-free!

A few months down the road, Susie surprised herself. After putting the decision on the back burner, she returned to the possibility of the breast augmentation and decided that she wanted the surgery after all. Not because she was disfigured or unlovable, but because she now saw it as a gift to herself: a procedure that would help her put the cancer behind her once and for all and feel more whole in her body. She felt grateful to live in a time where such surgery was readily available to her.

Later that fall, after dropping her daughter off at college, Susie returned home to a wonderful new man in her life who tells her something she already knows: "You're beautiful!"

Susie's story is strong evidence that the industry of aging can be a blessing—when we use it thoughtfully and in a way that supports, rather than replaces, positive and compassionate feelings toward ourselves. It also shows us, in the words of author David Richo, that "our wounds are often the openings into the best and most beautiful parts of us."

The first story about the woman my sister knew in the gym is a painful one because it's so resonant. Most of us struggle with at least some measure of discomfort about the signs of getting older that plague us. Watching our hair gray and our skin become wrinkled or the years fly by on the calendar, we might all wish to stay as young, sexy, boundlessly energetic, and ache-and-pain-free as when we were twenty-one. But that's not the way it works. Life has its own terms and we get to decide whether to try to beat them or to deal with them straight up.

The industry of aging will be glad to give you as many procedures, creams, hair colors, and spa treatments as you're willing to pay for, of course. So the responsibility, ultimately, lies with each of us. Before we fork over one more dollar on products and procedures that will supposedly reverse or disguise the natural effects of aging, let's stop and ask ourselves why.

Is doing so in keeping with feelings of shame, despair, desperation, and inadequacy? Is it a temporary fix? An ego boost? Or is it something inspired by the love, compassion, and acceptance you're cultivating for yourself as you get older? To quote author Jim Selman, founder of The Eldering Institute, "The ego doesn't get older—which is why the anti-aging industry is so successful."

You have to decide for yourself. Thanks to the revelations of your self-audit and the new vision you've mapped out for your best possible future, you have some guideposts to make your way through difficult age-related challenges. The power to choose well, tools to improve how you're dealing with getting older, and newfound courage to make It happen are all within your reach.

THE NATURAL ORDER OF THINGS: A "PACKAGE DEAL"

The industry of aging isn't only a reflection of our obsession with youth. It's also a symptom of profound changes in the way we get older and die.

"Old age itself has changed," wrote Dr. Atul Gawande in his remarkable book *Being Mortal*, released in 2014. Dr. Gawande wrote about how the experience of old age has transformed from a communal, multigenerational one—in which three generations regularly lived under a single roof—to a solitary experience that happens largely in an institutional setting surrounded by teams of medical professionals.

Modern US healthcare treats old age as a malady and death as a condition to be avoided at all costs (no matter the age or condition of the patient). Dr. Gawande gracefully reminds us that old age is *not* a malady—even as rapidly advancing medical technology is employed every single day to keep people from the natural processes of decline and death. Of course, it's predetermined that each of us will one day pass away. But that's hardly mentioned anywhere, by anyone, in polite conversation.

Our culture has become profoundly age- and death-phobic. We shy away from talking openly about these subjects; they are treated as embarrassing and as relevant only to those who are immediately and directly affected. The multibillion-dollar industry of aging has grown out of this cultural phenomenon—and then has helped to fuel it, by seemingly promising a fountain of youth.

We sanitize death. We have meticulous strategies for not dealing with it or addressing it at all. But more and more, and especially as baby boomers hit their golden years, there are so many of us dealing with aging and illness that we can't put it off any longer.

We are beginning to see the enormous problems with all this repression. Because we've turned the universal facts of aging and death into taboo subjects, we now feel isolated when we face them. Instead of collectively opting for denial, we could use the process of aging and facing death as powerful catalysts for getting to know ourselves as we are—and taking better care of ourselves. We'll miss out on that opportunity—unless we start to open ourselves to what we've previously considered taboo.

And that's why, in my workshops and coaching sessions, I approach this topic by emphasizing the "package deal" of life.

What do I mean by "package deal?"

Each of us is born into an imperfect world, to imperfect parents, with an imperfect body. As we grow, we learn that for every joy, there is a sorrow; for every blessing, there is a setback. This imperfect world is filled with gifts and miracles, but there is also hardship, suffering, and adversity.

Life is the package deal—the good, the bad, and the in-between.

Our challenge is to reconcile the "package." Amidst all the facets of life, we must learn to savor and recognize, experience and cherish the blessings. But we also must learn to deal with the unwelcome losses, changes, and challenges. And one of the most daunting obstacles in accepting life's package deal is the fear of what will become of us in the time leading up to, and after, life's natural conclusion.

The industry of aging has seemed to promise us a different kind of deal. With faith in their product or service, we can have half the package—only the good, only the beauty, only the joy, only *life*—without anything sad, bad, or ugly, without unhappiness or decline, and without death. That's not just absurd, it's dangerous.

In this culture that hides from, denies, and avoids the very facts of aging and death, we often hear a powerful negative message when we experience even the slightest signs of decline: that it's time to fold up the tent. Our value as human beings is diminishing. Having gone out of season, we're being relocated from Nordstrom to Nordstrom Rack.

Without knowing it, and oftentimes well before we're truly sick, we buy into these messages—and devalue ourselves. We no longer look, feel, or act like the world around us wants us to look, feel, and act. We're no longer on the upward trajectory that used to substantiate our worth and existence. Our "kids" are now adults occupied in their own busy lives. As these changes happen, we may, consciously or unconsciously, start to feel that we're no longer useful, that we no longer serve a purpose. And we slowly start to shut down the burners that are our life force.

Take a moment to consider whether you've been sending your mind, body, or spirit "shut-down" messages (or are sending them to an aging parent). Have you stopped going on the morning walks you used to love? Have you given up activities like dancing, biking, book club, or travel that have always been such a rich source of fun and joy? Have you stopped taking care of certain areas of your life or health, thinking to yourself, what's the point?

These changes might seem benign, but they act as subtle message to our subconscious: "Begin to pack up the tent."

There *is* a time of life for packing your bags and winding things down. I'm proud to say that I've had the honor and privilege of helping some great people pass on from this world, some of them long before their time. Whether we are worn down by years or ravaged by diseases like ALS or Alzheimer's, there *is* a time to let go.

What's deeply important to the process of courageous aging is that you set the terms for yourself. Stop buying into the subliminal messages of a culture that devalues you as you get older. Stop listening to what other people say you should do. Tune in to yourself and set your own (life-affirming rather than negating) terms.

It's important to note here that an entire book could be written about the differences between men and women when it comes to matters of age. Ask a female news anchor or actress like my friend Kimberley. Or an aspiring executive like my cousin Janie. They will tell you about the harsh double standards that still exist in our world. But you can also ask my buddy Danny, a fifty-six-year-old construction worker, whether the drop in his "market value" (losing work to younger men) affects how he feels about his age. None of us lives in a vacuum. We need to resist and reject society's prescriptions and prejudices about being a man or being a woman in favor of what's best for us as individuals.

Perhaps you're looking forward to slowing down a little after decades of being frenetically busy—and that's wonderful. You'll finally have time to take your foot off the gas pedal and feel a greater sense of ease about each day. You may choose to spend more quality time with your children and grandchildren. It might be the perfect time to begin fulfilling bucket-list travel adventures or staycations with your partner. The ability to simply stop and smell the roses, or to look in your spouse's, child's, or aging parent's eyes and tell them how much you love them, can enhance the quality of your life in ways you never imagined.

At the same time, it's important to negotiate making some very personal changes that benefit only you. I call this "good selfish." Do you wish you could do some long-awaited travel but find yourself making excuses that it's too late, or that your body can't handle it? Or giving up on your arthritic knees when your heart is aching to play golf with a few buddies during the week? Or doing something outlandish like taking a class in genomics with a Nobel Prize-winning visiting professor at a local university?

Go back to the vision that you've crafted for yourself. *That's* your road map. A new template for a new season of life. If you dream of biking through France as part of this new season of life, give a gift to your future self by going out for morning walks each day to keep yourself limber for the adventures ahead.

The package deal of life affirms life in *all* its phases, whereas the socially sanctioned industry of aging tells us to look like a "forever young" twenty-year-old or else to pack it in. Being able to embrace life as a package deal is an honest reminder that we get older, year by year. We are a work in progress and that's OK. Courageous living and aging is an invitation to live boldly— whatever that might mean to you—all the days of your life.

Breaking old habits of denial and embracing life as a package deal frees us to enjoy life as never before. Dealing with the seemingly unavoidable aches and pains of getting older, from bad knees to broken hearts, presents a different kind of challenge. Let's now explore effective ways of meeting, overcoming and even surrendering to those kinds of challenges.

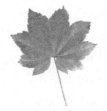

Chapter 7

PARTS AND SERVICE: I AM NOT MY ACHES AND PAINS

Gratitude unlocks the fullness of life. It turns what we have into enough.

—Melody Beattie

A while back, as I was doing my usual morning hike and generally feeling pretty decent in my then sixty-four-year-old body, there was an excruciating *POP*—and I came to a halt. Later at the doctor I would learn that I'd torn the tendons in my ankle.

After getting examined and bandaged—and elevated and iced, and bandaged again—I was told that the rehab for this kind of an injury was tricky. Most depressingly, I was told that it might not be wise for me to hike the trails any longer. Having had career-ending ankle surgery at age nineteen after making the all-star high school basketball team, I knew what was ahead. I'd have to patiently count the days until my cast came off, mind each step in order to keep from reinjuring it, and learn a whole new way of walking.

I was devastated by this setback to my otherwise vigorous life. I had always thought of myself as being in very good health for a guy my age. I'd bring guys ten year younger than me on my hikes and have to slow down when they were going uphill. This injury seemed to change all that: gimping around on crutches for several weeks, I felt old and weak. And the joke I'd been telling about "not dying of anything I know of" no longer seemed so funny.

I was so afraid of reinjuring myself that I moved very slowly and stiffly. Soon my hip began to hurt. The pain and the danger of that ankle collapsing strained other parts of my body. And for the second time in my life, I felt extremely fragile and like I was falling apart at the seams.

In the depressing and disheartening weeks after my accident, I "became" my aches and pains. I was so accustomed to feeling strong and to being self-reliant that being as helpless and debilitated as I was sent me into a tailspin. I didn't like this old guy with the broken wheel and worried that I would never be able to be myself again.

It turns out that both injuries and depression are pretty common bedfellows for guys my age. Our bodies just aren't as strong as they once were. Routine activity—like my morning hike on steep and uneven trails—often leads to injury. When we do get injured or sick, even the fittest and highly resourceful amongst us can spiral down into depression. Helplessness can start to creep in where we previously felt an affirming self-reliance. Losing any degree of independence is disheartening, and we are not accustomed to feeling so vulnerable.

Oddly enough, these kinds of physical changes can be some of the most difficult for those who previously felt the most self-reliant. I'd had great luck over the years hiking some of the most beautiful trails in North America several times a week. I thought it would go on forever. And then I got hurt. We can wait for a crisis before we step back and look at our expectations. Or we can learn to manage them accordingly by doing regular reality checks. Understanding what we're most attached to about ourselves—and where we may be holding on when it's time to let go—can help us recalibrate and manage our expectations.

MANAGING EXPECTATIONS AND EGOS

We're only human! Feeling weak and embarrassed about the inevitable changes in our bodies and minds (as though we failed the Jack Lalanne or Grandma Moses test), probably means we've set unreasonable expectations for ourselves and that we're holding ourselves to a standard that may no longer be attainable. It's one thing to start painting, like Grandma Moses, in our late seventies and make life an adventure. It's another to go paddle boarding on your eightieth birthday and break your pelvis. How and where we set our expectations, or shift them, including those tainted by society's antiquated double standards for men and women, is critical.

As uncomfortable as it may be, a reality check right now could be a helpful intervention. Most of us have gotten used to going for an annual physical. Exams are moments of truth where we get to see in very concrete ways how our bodies are changing. Guys joke about their prostate exams ("I asked my doctor why he was using two fingers and he told me, 'To get a second opinion.'") and women kid around about the trials and tribulations of menopause.

So why not a reality check to help us reset our expectations about the natural changes we all go through?

Stop and consider the natural trajectory of the human body. The wear and tear on our two hands, hard miles on our feet, relentless problem-solving of our minds, pumping of our hearts, churning of our stomachs, and timely elimination of waste all take their toll. Rather than show our bodies gratitude for the infinite ways they serve us, many of us elect to torture ourselves by comparing our current state to our younger selves. That's not just unhelpful; it's cruel. And it can be hazardous.

Imagine that your best friend has suffered an injury and that her recovery is going slower than expected. Would you criticize her by telling her that her thirty-five-year-old self would have bounced back by now? Of course not! Or would you embarrass a close relative who is struggling to remember the name of an old movie by commenting, "Having a senior moment?" Or would you egg on your older sister, a former cheerleader, when she comes to your Advanced Hot Yoga class and is just about to contort her 55-year-old body into pigeon pose with a "What's the matter girl? Not as easy as it looks, is it?" And yet we think nothing of lobbing such criticisms and admonitions at ourselves.

So give yourself the gift of stepping back from your present circumstances, whatever they may be. Remind yourself that you're in this new season of life and that it brings with it the good right along with the crappy—that's the package deal. And then take this opportunity to consider what you need to say or do to treat yourself with kindness and respect. Never has it been more important to take genuinely good care of yourself. Or to get your ego out of the way.

In my own recovery from an injury that felt both minor and cataclysmic, I became more mindful of taking good care of myself. As my ankle healed, I taped it up for extra strength and got myself a brand new pair of hiking boots with beefy ankle support. When the doctor gave me a set of exercises to strengthen the muscles that had weakened during my recovery, I vowed to do them religiously. I'm fighting my way back to the trail—even as I also recognize that I will never be exactly the same as I was. I will be a step slower and a tad more cautious. And that's OK.

In my own attempt to age courageously, and with the help of a wonderful physical therapist named Stephanie, I learned how to view my injury, as well as the general aches and pains of aging, as useful reminders of the very thing that our age-biased, death-phobic culture always seeks to deny: that I'm merely mortal. A torn ankle may appear unrelated to mortality. And certainly modern medical science, as I mentioned in the last chapter with respect to Dr. Gawande's book *Being Mortal*, will probably try to keep me going at least into my nineties with knee and hip replacements, laser therapy, and injections to regrow frayed cartilage and tendons.

But in fact, our small aches and pains are gentle (and sometimes not-so-gentle) reminders that everything changes. And that we are here on earth as part of a package deal. They're a reminder to be kind to ourselves, remember we're only human, and continue our work on this path of courageous living and aging—because it takes all the courage and strength we have!

I also discovered, embedded in the vulnerability of this relatively small accident, a connection to the family tragedy I spoke of earlier. It always amazes me how something that happened over twenty years ago can be awakened like this.

THE GREATEST LOSS—AND
EVENTUALLY, FINDING GRATITUDE

Like most stories of this nature, mine began on a seemingly normal evening. I had just walked in the door from picking my mother up at the airport and heard the phone ringing in my office. It was a mom whose daughter was also on the Semester at Sea program with our daughter, Jenna, asking if I knew about "the bus accident." After telling me "some of the kids were hurt pretty badly," there was a long pause, followed by, "And that one of those kids was Jenna." Sensing the worst, I fell to my knees. I was later told by my younger daughter, Stefie, that I had cried out, "Nooooooooooo. Please God, noooooooo."

My life as I knew it ended in that instant. Minutes later, I received a call from the US Embassy in India telling me our 21-year-old daughter had, in fact, died along with three other girls on a bus not far from the Taj Mahal.

To say that I was shattered doesn't express the depth or magnitude of what it was and has been like to lose Jenna. As I walked outside gasping for air, I knew that my life had changed forever. Strangely, at the same time I was searching the night sky for signs of my daughter, I also felt her right beside me. And I "heard" Jenna's voice. Not with my ears, the way I normally hear people speak. But in some other way. Maybe I was so distraught that I was hallucinating. Maybe I had slipped into another dimension of reality. But I "heard" my daughter Jenna speak to me. "Dad, it's not about you," she said in a tone that was intimately familiar. I had never had someone speak directly to my heart in that way, nor was that something I would have thought in a million years to say to my unspeakably distraught self.

Where was this coming from? Was there some part of my higher self that was now stepping in to guide me through this unimaginable tragedy? Was I summoning wisdom from within my own unconscious mind? Or imagination? Or was this coming *to* me? Was my daughter, now an angel, being my guiding light in a moment of utter darkness? Were these God's words? Or God's hand on my heart?

I didn't know.

What I did know was that I was heartbroken beyond words. My daughter's life, and her gloriously promising future, had been lost to her. And my life as I knew it had ended. As I stood in the ashes of ruin, my sorrow gave way to rage. I wanted to spit in the face of the universe. "How could you have let this happen?" I railed at God. "Tell me!" I had always believed in a spiritual being who was out there watching over my life and especially my children. Now I saw God as a negligent casting director who had either fallen asleep on the job or somehow made the decision that it was OK for my beautiful daughter to die.

After these first waves of raw sorrow and rage began to pass, I looked up to the sky and asked Jenna, "What now?"

Once again, I heard her voice.

"What now? More nows, Daddy," she answered instantaneously. *More nows?*

Where did this voice come from? Jenna had died hours earlier on the other side of the world, and yet she was speaking to me. Was I going crazy? (I've told countless bereaved parents "going crazy is the only sane response to losing a child.") Or was my daughter, now an angel, trying to tell me something. After a period of silence, Jenna's assurance, "I'm someplace more amazing than anything you can possibly imagine. And I'm OK, Daddy," allowed me to start breathing again and I walked inside.

In the months to come, I reflected on those moments. And there were more of them. Had I become psychotic and delusional in my desperation? Was this a response to the deepest despair I had ever felt?

I saw in that unfiltered moment that experiences like this are matters of faith; I did not know anything for certain, but I bet my faith that this was actually Jenna's voice. And in *hearing* her voice speaking out to me so lovingly and clearly, I chose to believe that my daughter was OK, that I'd be reunited with her one day, and that her hand would be reaching out to me when my time came.

As the days and weeks unfolded, what had happened slowly became the very core of my faith. We make a choice about what we believe, and we put our hearts and souls into that choice. And though we can never prove what we are experiencing with 100 percent certainty, it becomes our reality. And in that way our faith is that which gives us great comfort and allows us to experience the love that never dies.

Of course, having faith and coping with loss does not mean that we stop being sad. Or angry. Faith does not stop us from searching for greater truth and understanding. Or from learning. Faith allows us our moments of doubt, despair, and unknowingness. And we use these things to go even deeper. Giving myself permission to break down and cry on Jenna's birthday or to ride tidal waves of sorrow on days when missing her feels unbearable allows me to see I'm still grieving and gives me a constructive, healthy outlet for my sorrow. I have learned to accept that I will be triggered when I see a girl with her hair or find out that one of her friends just had a child or is a VP at Google. Indeed, those kinds of feelings may never go away. To hide, deny, reject, or resist giving them expression is to deny my humanity. And my enduring love.

I was forty-seven when Jenna passed. And in the years since, I've had the honor and privilege of working with people in the throes of trauma and tragedy. As I've turned gray and aspired to face my own aging in a courageous manner, I've begun to help others do the same. There are curiously striking similarities between losing a loved one and growing older. Grieving the loss of our younger self can bring up many of the same feelings as grieving the loss of someone we love. Sorrow, fear, and anger are natural, normal responses to any kind of significant loss. Both are momentous parts of the package deal. And in both, even as we grieve, we must somehow summon courage to prevail.

Indeed, I believe we define ourselves by how we respond in times of crisis. The kind of transition we make, or fail to make, to a new and unfamiliar normal requires newfound courage. History books are filled with colossal triumphs and failures that shape personal destinies and define the nobility or demise of the world's religions, its leaders, and its nations. And so it is today as we face the crises of violence, poverty, and global warming that threaten our very existence.

Twenty years after Jenna's death, I continue to feel sorrow that my daughter's life was lost to her and those who loved her. At the same time, I feel eminently grateful. Far worse than losing Jenna is to never have had her in my life for twenty-one miraculous and joyful years. I have learned to hold that gratitude right alongside the bottomless sorrow of her death. Of course, I wanted it all for Jenna. The full ride. But it was not to be. I do my best to focus on the gift of her life. In my work with the parents whose children were murdered in Newtown, Connecticut, I am reminded that they only had their children for five or six short years. I had Jenna for twenty-one glorious years. I am eternally grateful for that.

And so, even as aging brings unwelcome fear and sorrow, aches and pains, you might try holding your sorrow together with a sense of gratitude. They may seem strange bedfellows in life's package deal, but they tend to balance each other out.

Taking time to consider what you feel grateful for, calling up that feeling of deep appreciation and really taking it in is something you can do right now. Whether you write it down, place a spontaneous phone call, spread the love by feeding a homeless family, or sit in silence thanking a higher power, the expression of gratitude is perhaps one of the most healing, life-affirming things you can do.

Gratitude is also the antidote for the fear and resentment we so often feel when it comes to death. In the midst of feeling grateful for the blessings in our lives, we gain bargaining power with these unsettling emotions. "Sure it sucks that I'm going to die," a sixty-year-old client of mine told me before he passed, "but look at all good stuff I got to do while I was here. My wife. Kids. Company. And yeah, listening to Andrea Bocelli sing. I am a very lucky man." Accepting life's package deal is a tough proposition, especially when we've received final notice that the end is near. Giving expression to our gratitude helps us balance out the bad stuff and take some more baby steps toward a peaceful reconciliation.

THE LOVE THAT NEVER DIES

Perhaps you, too, have lost someone you love and were shattered. Or you have suffered a living loss, where the past, present, and/or future with someone you love has been "lost" to estrangement, alcoholism, addiction, divorce, or a debilitating illness. You feel utterly helpless. Powerless. And you have nowhere to turn. There is no greater pain than that of love that can't be expressed. Someone falls terminally ill, dies, relapses, or leaves us. And the love has nowhere to go. When the expression of love is thwarted, we implode. For this reason, I believe it's important to find the part of the relationship that does go on: the love that never dies.

I feel fortunate to have heard Jenna's voice right from the very moment I learned of her passing. This helped me see the possibility of maintaining my relationship with her even though it would take place in something I have come to call a "spiritual realm." And I've done exactly that, all these years. I even joke with audiences: "Yes, I talk to the dead," when teaching grief literacy. Asking if there's "anybody from the 'thought police' in the audience who might want to disbar, excommunicate, or throw me in a psych ward" brings laughter. But it also sets the stage for making it safe to have the critically important conversation (usually reserved for psychics and mediums) about the love than never dies.

The possibility of maintaining a loving relationship with someone who has passed away might seem impossible, but my experience—and the experiences of so many others who have suffered such a loss—suggests otherwise. Love after loss is a matter of what you choose to believe or your faith. And it is best spoken about with humility and grace.

Your spiritual self is tuned to a different frequency than your rational, evidence-based, scientific self. And that's OK. There's nothing to prove or disprove. There's just what you choose to believe, what you hope for, and where you place your bet when it comes to the true nature of things.

When we lose a loved one, we no longer have access to the physical, three-dimensional relationship that we've always had. In its stead, we have the choice to convert that physical relationship into a spiritual one. Over time, as we move forward in our lives with no choice but to endure the physical absence of our loved one, we can begin to cultivate a connection with that person on a spiritual level. This can take many forms. You might simply feel that person in your heart. They might be fully alive and vivid in your memory. Maybe they're situated only in your imagination: You see them in the here and now, joining you as your life continues to unfold. Or maybe they're present in what you (and I) have come to know as a spiritual realm.

If you already have an active faith life, this type of relationship may be familiar to you. If not, this idea may seem strange or feel uncomfortable. Regardless of your beliefs, though, being grateful for what you did have and cultivating a spiritual relationship is a powerful way of dealing with the loss of a loved one. And staying connected by the love that never dies can actually allow it to grow even stronger.

If we met, you might notice the moonstone necklace I wear around my neck. In very small letters, around the moonstone is engraved the word "HINENI." In Hebrew that means "I am here."

A new friend gave me this moonstone after a speech about the paradox of Jenna being both gone *and* always here, right beside me. "The highest form of understanding love and loss," I had explained, "is in understanding the paradoxical nature of life." Going from an *either/or* to a *both/and* way of seeing things allows us to experience our loved ones as here (hineni) and gone. We come to know and compassionately accept ourselves as both broken and whole. And as our new lives unfold, we find them to be both bitter and sweet.

As humans, we love, and we lose. We feel both old and forever young as the timeless, undying essence of us, and the essence of our loved ones, lives on. Allowing both our brokenness and wholeness, seeing them as parts of us, frees us to move forward and write new chapters of life.

MOVING
FORWARD

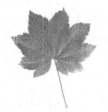

Chapter 8
REIMAGINING THE
FUTURE: THE NEW OLD

I'm choosing happiness over suffering, I know I am. I'm making space for the unknown future to fill up my life with yet-to-come surprises.
—Elizabeth Gilbert

don't know where to turn."

That's what Stella, a grief-stricken, forty-four-year-old woman told me over the phone as she contemplated attending one of my talks on resilience at a local women's conference. After twenty-two years of "turbulent" marriage, Stella's husband had told her that he'd fallen in love with someone else—someone *younger*—and that he wanted a divorce. "I'm still in shock," she told me, "and I just can't stop crying."

In a great leap of faith, Stella came to my talk. Although she couldn't imagine finding her way out of the sorrow and betrayal she felt, she decided it was time to learn about resilience and how to channel her pain into something positive. Stella was determined to face down her crisis and draw up a hopeful new plan for her future. Little did she realize that there was a major roadblock standing in her way.

She was brutally honest when she stood up during the Q & A period following my talk and confessed, "For the first time in my life, I feel old. And disposable." Stella was drowning in her own self-loathing for not being younger, sexier, or "spontaneous" enough to keep her husband's interest.

As it turned out, she was in good company at the workshop, where men and women from age forty to seventy openly discussed the critical and even cruel ways that they had judged and devalued themselves after a setback. Many people, including Stella, had never stepped back from their interior critical voices and experimented with voices of self-compassion. Nor had they realized how much Kool-Aid they had drunk over the years when it came to aging.

My talk on resilience turned into a group awakening. Quoting a famous movie line in the film *Network*, one woman stood up and shouted, "I'm mad as hell and I'm not going to take this anymore," as wild laughter broke out. For the first time in a long time, Stella began to feel hopeful. "Hey, I'm only forty-four years old. I've got my whole life ahead of me," she declared as we wound down and gathered up our things to leave the conference. Stella had begun to take back her power. And her future. Only *she* would be the one to determine her own value, decide whether she was beautiful, and choose how to move forward.

Stella signed on for a few private coaching sessions after my talk. With an enthusiasm that would have been hard to imagine just a few weeks before, Stella started drafting new plans for her life: Having been a talented potter in her twenties, Stella signed up for a ceramics class to revitalize her love of art. She had also started looking into moving into an apartment in downtown San Diego, because she loved the vibrancy of the city. She would be within walking distance of museums, live music and theatre, sporting events, and a variety of things that her husband had never been interested in. Stella also decided that she wanted a new look for this new version of herself and found a great new hair stylist.

At the tender age of forty-four, Stella had just wholeheartedly embraced something I call "The New Old." You heard what I had to say about the myths of graceful aging back in Chapter 3. These myths are short-lived stories designed to placate us. They sidestep the real challenges of getting older and keep us in a comatose state of avoidance. In direct contrast to this passive, compliant mindset, The New Old is a state of awakening. Dealing straight up with things that make us feel old, as well as the ones that leave us feeling ageless, we realize that both are real. Paradoxically, we are getting old and we are ageless. Both are true. And this is what makes us human. We do have a choice about which side of our nature to feed—and what to make of our days. Whether we prefer to relive the past or live in the present and create the future, become lesser or better version of ourselves, be passive observers or engaged participants is ultimately our choice. The New Old is not an overly simple, economically driven slogan for turning seventy into the new fifty. It is a code for living and aging that guides us to enjoy the (actual) best parts of our lives.

Another great example of people whose lives were transformed by embracing The New Old is a sixty-two-year-old firefighter named Brad whose wife, Ellie, had died of ALS.

After Ellie passed away, Brad was understandably lost. His long and happy marriage had ended after years of nursing his wife through her illness. Having taken off work for several months and been his wife's caregiver, going to sleep and getting up each day was a challenge, as was filling the empty space in his day. After attending a Compassionate Workplace program I gave at his fire station, he slowly returned to work. The guys at the fire station could not have been more supportive. Several of them even donated their sick days to extend his bereavement leave.

Halfway through the first year, Brad even began accepting dinner invitations from friends and getting out more. Facing the prospect of getting to know someone new, however, was terrifying. Despite his wife's loving assurance that he not spend the rest of his life alone, his years as a caretaker had drained him, and he had shut down in most every possible way. For the longest time, he didn't know if it was even possible to share this next phase of life with another companion. And he stayed in his cave.

But a little over a year after Ellie's passing, he was ready. When someone set him up with a woman from church whose husband had also died, he accepted the invitation. Even though that date went horribly, it was the icebreaker he needed. "We would have killed each other," he joked with me. Brad kept meeting women and going on dates for the next six months until he met a special woman named Kirsten.

Kirsten was a perfect match for Brad. As they grew closer, Kirsten honored how wonderful his relationship with Ellie had been, how much he continued to grieve her loss, and accepted that Ellie would always have a place in his heart. Brad accepted and appreciated her loving support, slowly allowing himself to fall in love again. The one place Brad had trouble adjusting was in bed. The pressure he put on himself to perform, and the intense emotions of holding another woman's naked body in his arms proved overwhelming.

Like Stella, Brad had become attached to the idea of how he thought he *should* be. And what he thought he should be able to do. He ruthlessly compared himself to the "sex machine" he was at thirty and underestimated the lingering effects of losing Ellie in such an excruciatingly painful way.

Yet when he and Kirsten started talking about all this, Brad began feeling 100 percent better. Seeing the ways Ellie's illness and death had devastated him, and how his inability to perform was not a sign of old age, he felt relieved. And then guess what happened?

Going through this with Kirsten not only affirmed his confidence and trust in her, it helped him to see more of what he wanted for his future. "I want to be able to cry when I need to and slowly learn to enjoy myself again," he told me, breaking a smile. "I'm sixty-two and I've been through hell, but I feel younger today that I have in fifteen years."

The New Old is about letting go of myths, age-related fears, and insecurities. Welcoming in the wiser, more compassionate, and confident version of himself was a triumph for Brad and the new woman in his life, who had grown to adore him. Going through this kind of transition, navigating our way from the world of myths to realities, looks a little different for everyone. Each one of us faces different kinds of challenges. And being a man or a woman; black, white, or brown; rich or poor; single or married can present its own additional challenges. But living mindfully in the realm of The New Old has its benefits.

PERKS OF THE NEW OLD:

These New Old benefits come from following the tenets for courageous living and aging described in this book:

- awakening to psycho-spiritual insights in the middle and later stages of life
- letting go of old baggage, fears, resentments, and insecurities and accept life as the package deal
- finding a path to newfound freedom, peace, and security
- being present and compressing (spreading out the reaches of) time rather than living in the past and/or future (i.e., "fleeting" time)
- strengthening our relationships with our loved ones
- generating a "pay it forward" spirit
- facing into, rather than avoiding, issues of aging that arise in ourselves, our families, and our communities and society
- exploring our place in the greater scheme of things and making peace with death

Choosing the ones that resonate with you and then weaving them into your daily routines and practices is a winning formula.

THE GREATEST ASPIRATION OF THEM ALL

"I just faced my own mortality head on," my friend Natasha Josefowitz, a vivacious ninety-year-old, recently wrote in her column for the *La Jolla Village News*. "A few days ago I met my new twin great-grandsons—all of four months old—and realized I will not know them as teenagers! They will have to see me on old DVDs, which may in fact not be playable by then."

As she cradled her great-grandsons, Natasha could have felt saddened and defeated when facing her own mortality. Instead she used it as an opportunity to imagine the future, and to reflect on how she wanted to spend her nineties:

I will miss so much fun like everyone having driverless cars and Amazon packages flying in via drones through an open window. I will probably not get to print my 3-D sandwiches in what will be a common household appliance, nor use a robot to clean my house, nor be privy to dozens of other not-as-yet discovered wonders that will retool our brains, change our DNAs and make our lives easier (hopefully).

On the other hand, I was born on a street paved with cobblestones; milk [was] delivered in glass bottles with the cream rising to the top, by means of a horse-drawn carriage. A large block of ice was brought to the house to be placed in the aptly named icebox to drip quietly into a tray at the bottom. Doctors made house calls and now do the same via Skype.

Things that were not invented yet are obsolete now—like pantyhose, VHSs, and electric typewriters.

I, indeed, am part of a generation in transition. . . .

Ninety years from now the world will be as different, if not more so, than ninety years ago.

Reflecting on the ways that technology has changed for the better, Natasha found a kernel of wisdom for her own best possible future:

I like the unknown people who want to be my friends on Facebook, or my columns reaching untold numbers on Huffington Post. I like the easy way of reaching friends by e-mails and texts, receiving a photo from a grandchild within minutes of it being taken, sending kisses via Skype or FaceTime to a grandbaby. I like the whirlwind of my life, but not the mass of papers that seem to copulate endlessly, not ever allowing me to be caught up. My file cabinets are bulging with information I have not looked at in years, with the mindset that it might be needed again someday. Some day . . . some day I will become a minimalist and live in an environment devoid of clutter. In the meantime, I really should take everything out of my freezer and see what is still there as leftovers from a party too long ago. As long as I'm doing that, I should also give away all the shoes with heels that I shall never wear again.

So, dear reader, you can see where my musings of my own mortality have taken me: declutter—simplify my life to make room for whatever will come next.

Natasha is a role model, and an ambassador for The New Old. At ninety, she's never felt more comfortable with who and what she is. What's more, embedded in this piece of her writing is another deeply important aspect of The New Old: the concept psychologist Erik Erikson dubbed *generativity*.

According to Erikson, generativity is a felt sense of responsibility and concern for the next generation. It arises through a feeling of optimism for the future and for humanity at large. In this, too, Natasha is a role model; she's spending her golden years helping the rest of us see the continuity between the old world that she was born into, our modern twenty-first-century world, and the future that's ahead for our great-grandchildren. Natasha wants to build bridges between the generations, so that we feel more connected to, and responsible for, those who come after us.

There's not enough "seventh generation" mentality at work in our society, and we cannot afford short-sightedness about our environment, safety and security, or health. Very much connected to this notion of generativity, the "seventh generation" credo was established by the Iroquois tribe and its belief in the importance of planting a metaphorical tree that will grow tall enough to give shade to our children and to their children and their children. Indeed, it is an elegant way of regarding our responsibility as human beings to not leave the world—or at least our small corner of it—in horrific disarray.

The seventh generation mentality leads to these questions: Have we done *our part* to create some peace in this world? What gifts have we left behind that will benefit others after we are no longer?

You might not have expected to find this sort of question in a book about courageous aging: wrinkle creams and memory loss, yes, but the seventh generation credo, probably not. And yet this is an integral part of The New Old ethic for cultivating gratitude and paying it forward. As we courageously embrace our aging selves, we can become hopelessly self-involved or positively clear about the *common good* and what really matters.

Some of us, like my friend Paul, find ourselves in a state of utter despair over the state of our nation and world. Fearing the inclusive "global" ideals he fought for over his lifetime are going to be replaced by exclusive, "nationalistic" ones, he feels outraged and powerless. "My legacy of leaving the world a better place is in serious jeopardy," he confessed, adding, "I may not be the twenty-seven-year-old law student who fought for civil and human rights back in the day but I will fight for what I believe in as long as I have breath in me."

We can hoard everything we own or we can declutter our lives. We can stockpile things, as in ancient Egypt, or learn to let go of them. And we can disengage and turn away from what's happening in our world, or fight valiantly for what we believe in.

The people we love matter. We matter. Our communities and nation matter. And the legacy that we leave behind matters.

So when the moment is right for you, take some time to consider your own position about all this. How would you like to make a better tomorrow for the seventh generation?

And as you turn toward these larger questions, you're likely to find that your former fears and insecurities will probably begin to fade a bit (even though they may never entirely disappear). As they do, you will likely feel something inside of you shift, giving way to a higher calling. Paying your heightened sense of gratitude and fullness forward is the most powerful part of The New Old.

My daughter Jenna was only fifteen when she adopted an adage that originated among the Lakota Sioux—and yet it embodies this very spirit of fullness. "Dad," she said to me one day, bright and smiling, "there's an old Native American saying that goes: Today is a good day to die!" I had such a beautiful day today with you and Mommy, Stefie, and my friend Pilar, that I think I understand what they mean. Today would be a good day to die!"

Yes, Jenna was wise beyond her years. She was an elder spirit in a girl's body. She saw the wisdom in making the days of our lives count for something to the point that we can say, "Today is a good day to die." For the Lakota Sioux, it meant that they were so present in each day, and so full of life, and they felt such deep connection to their loved ones, that death was nothing to fear. And all the good we had in this life would be paid forward. This is the highest aspiration of The New Old.

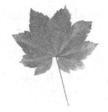

Chapter 9
PUTTING YOUR
HOUSE IN ORDER

The best thing about the future is that it comes one day at a time.

—Abraham Lincoln

This chapter is about getting your house in order—which can mean very different things to different people. Let's start with Joan's story.

"I'm a late bloomer," Joan told me at my most recent Courageous Aging workshop.

I soon learned what Joan meant by that. She had spent a lot of her life in the shadow of something her father had told her when she was a girl—and then, as a woman, took an enormously brave step to overcome it.

From the time Joan was eight, her dream was to be a veterinarian. She loved animals and she knew that she wanted to spend her life caring for them. She treasured that dream and pictured herself as an adult, spending her days helping dogs and cats to be healthy.

When her dad got wind of this, he sat her down and told her, "Girls don't go to college—and they sure don't become veterinarians."

Needless to say, Joan was crushed. She told me that, at that moment, her heart sank into her stomach—and stayed there for thirty-five years. Even as she picked another career and had a family of her own, Joan still fantasized about becoming a veterinarian, though she told no one about this dream.

Then Joan met one of the kindest human beings she'd ever encountered. And it changed her life. Alison was a hospice vet who had spent most of one Sunday with Joan's family as they said goodbye to their elderly Labrador. "Alison could not have been more loving with all of us—and under the very worst of circumstances," Joan told me. Alison was not only tender and compassionate, she was as skillful and devoted to her work as anyone Joan had ever witnessed. Although a part of her had died that day as her beloved dog slipped away, another part of her came back to life. Allison had awakened the dreams of an eight-year-old of becoming a vet. And that was the day she decided to go to veterinary school.

Within a month, Joan had talked it over with her husband and kids, applied to a local veterinary school, got accepted, and enrolled. When classes began a month later, Joan found that she wasn't just the oldest student, she was the same age as some of her fellow students' mothers. She knew that she could have let her age, or her father's beliefs about girls and women, stand in her way for her entire life. But she wasn't going to do that. She was finally going after her dream.

As Joan's experience makes clear, sometimes getting our house in order means deciding to do something that seems impossible at your age. It might involve pursuing a long-ignored dream, patching up a broken relationship, organizing your affairs so that you and your loved ones are prepared, or doing *all* of those things!

This process requires getting clear about what time it is in your life and what practical matters need to be handled for you to be at peace. And it requires old-fashioned elbow grease to face the areas of your life that you may have been avoiding. Or that have been too uncomfortable to address. Many of us delay the work of drafting a will or engaging in estate planning with an attorney. The same goes for stipulating who will make medical decisions for us when we can't make them for ourselves.

It's easy to postpone these things because we think there will always be more time and that there will be a better time than this one. Be forewarned: The buck stops here. And now. *This* is the time.

YOUR CHECKLIST FOR CLEANING HOUSE

Every time we put some element of our house in order—be it the handling of our finances, estate plan/will, business affairs, matters of the heart, or those affecting our family—we feel a sense of relief. No matter what happens now, we know those matters have been taken care of. We can breathe a sense of relief, kick back, and enjoy life knowing we've acted responsibly. This chapter goes through several of the most critically important "rooms" of your house, beginning with your personal life, so you can take charge and put your affairs in order. This is a gentle reminder to record your answers to these important questions by writing them out on a blank piece of paper in your notebook—or in the space provided in the Courageous Living and Aging booklet which is downloadable from www.kendruck.com.

Your Personal Life

- ☐ Do you feel good about the life you're leading today? If not, what changes would you like to make? (Remember that Joan started veterinary school in her forties!)
- ☐ If you're at a crossroads in your life, what are the choices before you? Which of these options is most likely to result in your health/happiness?
- ☐ What health and well-being, or lifestyle practices and changes, might you incorporate in order to remain mentally, physically, and spiritually vibrant?
- ☐ How might you do a better job of balancing out the parts of you that either push you too hard, or not hard enough, when it comes to retaining your (youthful) energy and enthusiasm?
- ☐ Do you feel good about the relationships you have with your family and friends? If not, what can you say and/or do to make them better? Which relationships need tending to?
- ☐ What do you want your loved ones to know after you're gone? Your wishes for/feelings towards them? Requests? Reminders?
- ☐ Do you plan on telling your loved ones these things? If so, how and when?

Your Medical, Financial, And Legal Life

- ☐ Have you created a will or trust and an estate plan with an attorney?
- ☐ If so, are they current and up to date?

- [ ] If not, what are you waiting for? What's holding you back?
- [ ] What would have to happen for you to get the names of a few competent and trustworthy attorneys you could work with on these matters?
- [ ] Have you chosen someone to make medical decisions for you if you can't make them for yourself? Have you provided instructions about what types of care you do and do not want? If not, the Five Wishes medical directive or something similar can provide clear instructions.
- [ ] Do you have a doctor whom you trust and who knows you well? If not, are you willing to find one and build a relationship with them/their staff?
- [ ] Have you left instructions, passwords, and legal and financial information in case of an emergency?
- [ ] Who can access your computer, phones, safe, etc., should you die? Do they currently have the means to do so?

• • • • •

Each of these areas is individually important, and together they add up to the peace of mind that you need and deserve in this new season of life.

Consider just the importance of having a doctor whom you know and trust. In her final years, having a loving and devoted doctor like "Dr. Bruce (Sachs)" by her side made all the difference for my mother. As I've gone through my fifties and sixties, my doctor, Dr. Lee Rice, and his wonderful staff at the Lifewellness Institute, have played a significantly greater part in my life.

After I injured my ankle last year, I confronted my own vulnerability. I also embraced the fact that I'm likely to become more susceptible to injury and illness. And that I need to put myself in better shape to prevent these kinds of things in the years ahead. I feel blessed to have an enormously competent and devoted physician like Dr. Rice to turn to when I need him.

Completing a medical directive is also absolutely essential. In our modern age, medical staff often make heroic attempts to prolong life—even when that means the patient only lives for a couple of days and does so in a lonely hospital bed instead of at home surrounded by family. What matters most to you at the end? Give yourself and your loved ones the gift of communicating your wishes to someone who can realize them on your behalf.

START SMALL, GIVE THANKS, AND PAY IT FORWARD

You might feel a sense of trepidation in looking at these checklists. You may feel that there's too much to be done, or that there are family members who cannot be approached with such sensitive matters. While it's true that some fences cannot be mended, you owe it to yourself and your family to give it a shot, or, in the words of legendary songwriter John Lennon, to "give peace a chance." So start small. One conversation at a time. Soften your tone. And build from there. Summoning your courage one more time, decide which subjects can be addressed most easily. And do those first. Then, with that sense of momentum and newfound confidence, tackle one that's a little more challenging. Keep moving up the list. You might surprise yourself.

Having consulted with many families and family businesses over the years, I'm well aware of the difficulties that can arise. Sometimes we unknowingly open Pandora's box and all hell breaks loose. Stepping around minefields and long-held family conflicts of interest can be exhausting and even treacherous. Bringing in a family specialist to help you navigate these rough waters can turn emotionally charged conversations and misunderstandings into long-overdue and much-needed communication. Families who are able to put these kinds of issues on the table and deal with them are more likely heal old wounds, make amends, find forgiveness, and forge new understandings. The result—sound decision-making, new agreements, a house in order, and peace of mind—are well worth the investment.

You don't have to be a Benedictine monk to put your house in order. Benedictine monks start each day by considering it to be their last, and then they treat it as such as they move through the hours. For most of us, that's too extreme. You don't need to become morbid or hyper-spiritual in order to put your house in order. There's a balance to be found. In this process of courageous aging, you're acknowledging some of the realities of getting older, and you're tending to your affairs. Not only is this a proactive way of paying the good in your life forward, it's a means of preventing unnecessary hardship. In doing so, you're clearing away those nagging worries—so that you can turn your focus to the important business of living!

We are choosing to *bless* our lives. We're giving thanks for all the good that we've received, we're taking care of our relationships and ourselves in the face of the unknown, and we're unencumbering ourselves so that we can pay that good forward. This is what it means to make peace. And to leave *generosity of heart* as your legacy.

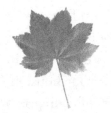

Chapter 10
IRREVERENT, VIBRANT, AND AUDACIOUS AGING

We must be willing to let go of the life we've planned, so as to have the life that is waiting for us.
—**Joseph Campbell**

Natasha Josefowitz, my beloved friend whose column about aging you read back in Chapter 8, is my role model for audacious aging. Natasha is more irreverent today than she was thirty years ago—when she was writing best-selling business books *and* poetry. Her story is an invitation for all of us to resist and refuse getting "old" by choosing to stay active, engaged, courageous, and curious.

In addition to writing her own weekly column, Natasha is the author of twenty books ("Twenty *so far*," she would add). She gives keynote speeches at conventions, writes for the *Huffington Post*, sits on eight committees and is pioneering a "buddy system" to help her ninety-year-old contemporaries become more engaged in activities that fill their lives with meaning. And as if all that weren't enough, she's working with gerontologists at the University of California on cutting-edge technology that can be most useful to aging populations. As a culture we have prevailing ideas about what it means to be ninety years old—and Natasha has laughed at all of them. "I'm doing the best work of my life," she told me recently.

At the same time, Natasha has become—by her own admission—a more loving, intimate, and centered version of herself. Sitting by the ocean at lunch not long ago, she squeezed my hand telling me how much she missed her late husband, Herman. And she teared up while talking joyfully about her grandkids. Natasha listened compassionately as I talked about how much I miss my "angel daughter," Jenna, and how happy I am for my "earth daughter," Stefie, whose relationship with her husband, Tony, is everything I would wish it to be.

Natasha is honest about her life's greatest sorrows and about the prospect of her own mortality—and then, she'll jot down some notes for her next column, post a picture to Facebook from her phone, and call a girlfriend to grab a burger and see a movie.

I want to be like her when I grow up! And you might be thinking the same thing. While there are no guarantees, this chapter enumerates a handful of strategies to help make you—and to help *keep* you—audacious so that you can enjoy whatever you consider to be your older years, be they your eighties, nineties, or one hundreds.

VIGOROUS IN BODY AND MIND, AUDACIOUS IN SPIRIT

For most of the last two decades, I've carried an extra thirty pounds on my frame. I love food (plus Ben and Jerry and sourdough bread have never once said no to me and they love me unconditionally) and I'm not able to work out the way I used to. I succeeded in losing weight a number of times, but it never lasted. Within a year, I was back to my former weight. Then, this year, something *clicked* inside of me. First, my knees spoke, "Ken, we hurt most all the time. You're now sixty-seven years old and we can't continue on this way." Next, it was my daughter, "Daddy, I want you around for a long time. Please take better care of yourself!" Then, I learned from genetic testing that I didn't have an "off switch" to tell me I was full. And so I would keep eating long past the point that was healthy. And finally, under the weight of all these things, something shifted deep inside of me. The rationalizations and denial I'd been using to justify my behavior no longer held water. It really hit me how all that extra weight was taking its toll on me and creating pain. I was at a serious choice point in my life. So I made a solemn decision to lose weight—and this time it was different.

Was it different because my father died of congestive heart failure when he was sixty-nine? I feel cheated out of the years I could have had with him, and, if for no other reason than being there for my daughter, Stefie, I want to live much longer than my dad.

My daughter was also committed to getting herself in better shape and asked, "Dad, would you do this with me?" I felt something in me leap to the challenge.

Six months and thirty pounds later, my creaky old knees are happier than they've been in twenty years. I'm getting all sorts of compliments and wearing beautiful shirts and sport jackets I haven't been able to put on in fifteen years. And with encouragement from my daughter and my fiancé, Lisette, I even went out shopping and bought some really sharp, slimmer-fitting duds to celebrate my new look.

Courageous Aging isn't a book about weight-loss strategies, but it *is* a book about choosing health—physical, emotional, and spiritual—as you get older. It means investing in yourself by actually taking the time to exercise instead of just promising you will in the future. Being better/smarter than that old version of Ken Druck who carried an extra thirty pounds means keeping company with the new Ken Druck, whose slimmer, spryer body sends the signal "live" to my brain.

Staying healthy as you turn fifty, sixty, or seventy means something different than it meant when you were thirty or even forty. I may still fantasize about putting on my old (musty and sitting in the back of a storage closet) soccer shoes and pads and playing just like I used to. It's been fifteen years since I suited up in soccer shorts, T-shirt with my team name and knee brace—and, frankly, I should throw them all away. My knees can no longer take the pounding. Accepting the reality that soccer isn't right for my body anymore, and letting go, is harder than I thought. I may not quite be ready yet to chuck my old gear, but I did go out and get myself some great new hiking shoes and an orange yoga mat. And as think about it all, I feel a warm sense of gratitude; I am very lucky to have played soccer for as long as I did, and, skipping off to a gentle yoga class, or to a sunset hike on the trails overlooking the ocean near my home, I have discovered new joy.

The returns on investment for staying active and moving our bodies— greater health and joy—are essential ingredients when it comes to our best possible future.

The same is true for good nutrition. The "right" foods and supplements, in all likelihood, may be different from when you were younger. Dr. Andrew Weil has a series of invaluable books, including *Healthy Aging: A Lifelong Guide to Your Well-Being*, that spell out a healthful diet tailored to the needs of an aging body.

Dr. Weil explains how certain foods (like refined carbohydrates, red meat, fried foods, and sugar-sweetened beverages) trigger or exacerbate inflammation and make it harder to combat conditions ranging from arthritic knees to heart disease or cancer. Meanwhile, other foods act as *anti-inflammatories*: leafy greens, tomatoes, blueberries, walnuts, olive oil, and others. Indeed, part of courageous aging is to leave behind the "unconditional love" and great taste we have come to crave in processed foods and choose foods that genuinely nourish our bodies. Sorry, Ben and Jerry. It's over!

Breakthrough research in neuropsychology has also been producing methods for keeping our brains healthy and sharp as we get older. To keep her brain active, Natasha told me she writes, speaks, and collaborates with scientists at UCSD. Those activities aren't possible for all of us, of course. Maybe for you it's scouring the Internet, doing crossword puzzles, taking a class at a local college, or joining a book club. Listening to or playing music, painting, or writing poetry also activate your brain and keep it sharp. The old saying "you can't teach a dog new tricks" is entirely wrong. Just ask John Assaraf, founder of NeuroGym, or any of the world's other leading neuroscientists and they will tell you, "Our brains are flexible and plastic and astonishingly powerful."

Amid all this physical and mental fitness, it's also important to take the time you need to rest and replenish. Good self-management means balancing rest and activity, getting a good night's sleep, taking breaks, coming up for air and making sure we have quiet time. Working with high-performing teams and giving talks on burnout prevention over the years, and then publishing *The Self-Care Manual*, have taught me the critical importance of finding balance as we get older. It means not pushing yourself when your body is saying no, learning to relax and unplug from the stream of daily activity. The moments we get to spend in quiet solitude, stillness, and silence also replenish and rejuvenate us when our batteries are low. And then, of course, treating ourselves, now and again, to some pampering—a deep-tissue massage, a spa day, a walk in nature, or, if you're adventurous, a yoga/meditation retreat, are great ways to recharge our batteries.

Kindness is not something we think about when talking in the same breath as irreverence, vibrancy, and audacity. But it plays a key role. Besides being audacious and irreverent, is there anything more important than being kind to yourself as a way of dealing with some of the unwelcome changes associated with aging?

Consider the situation of Amy, who has worked as an executive assistant to one of my best buddies, Ed, for twenty-five years. Over the years, Amy has assisted Ed, a well-known author and speaker, and is to a great degree responsible for his success. In all honesty, Ed would be lost without her and takes great pride in boasting, "Nothing slips through the cracks when Amy's on the case!" Recently, though, I got a call from Amy telling me she "didn't know where else to turn." "Something's happening to me, Ken. I can't seem to remember the names of people I've known for twenty minutes or twenty years anymore. I'm turning sixty-five next month and I'm really scared." I suggested that we take a few minutes to talk, and we did for the next hour.

"For God's sake, Ken, what's going on?" she asked. "Am I getting Alzheimer's?" I told her I didn't know, that I would also be scared if this was happening to me and would be glad to help her find out. Amy agreed to have her cognitive function assessed by a top-notch neurologist I recommended and made an appointment to get checked out. We also agreed that she'd stop attacking and discrediting herself for what was happening. And she would avoid dwelling on the worst possible explanation. Amy and I concluded that no matter what turned out to be causing her memory lapses, the most profoundly important thing she could do was be kind to herself.

The anti-aging properties of kindness and self-compassion have probably never been studied, but I would bet they will someday be proven effective. A wise friend of seventy-eight once told me he'd changed what he used to say to himself when looking in the mirror from a scathing, "Look at you! You old man!" to "Look at you! You handsome devil!"

And what about the anti-aging properties of humor? Sometimes, we have to be able to smile, shake our heads, laugh at ourselves, and joke about our circumstances. We take things so seriously and make the small stuff into a big deal. In reality, each of us is not even a tiny speck of dust on a planet that's actually a minuscule grain of sand flying through a vast, black universe. The first time it occurred to me how insignificant my fears and worries were in the larger scheme of things, I remember thinking, "I'm *an extra* in some intergalactic comedy!"

The ability to lighten up is a greater and greater asset as we get older. Taking a deep breath, letting our jaws and shoulder drop, and, for a moment, allowing the smallness of our existence be a source of perspective can calm a turbulent heart. So can treating yourself to a piece of dark chocolate, a slice of thin-crusted pizza, or a great romantic comedy.

CAUGHT UP IN THE IDENTITY TRAP

Whether you're retired, contemplating retirement, or certain that you never want to retire at all, an important part of audacious aging is to honor and appreciate the role that work has played in your life up until this point. And then begin to let it go.

We work to make money, of course. But we also work for other reasons. Many of us, for example, derive most of our sense of purpose and personal significance from our professional lives. The United States in particular has a very work-oriented culture, and we tend to define ourselves by what we do; indeed, "What do you do?" is one of the most common questions we ask when we meet someone new. Work also very often supplies us with our sense of self-esteem. And value. We may even feel that our dedication to work gives us a "hall pass" from having to perform in personal relationships, health and fitness, or community. No wonder so many of us take refuge in our jobs when other areas of our lives seem to be crumbling. And is it any wonder that such a great number of us who have been MIA from other parts of our lives dread the world of retirement?

RETIRING FROM RETIREMENT

So who will you be when you decide to retire from being a teacher, lawyer, executive assistant, salesperson, doctor, police officer, business owner, soldier, ten-time All Pro quarterback, or president of the United States of America? What do we call someone who doesn't "do" anything anymore? A retiree? For too many of us, retirement becomes a nightmare. We find ourselves lost and staring into the abyss. For others, it becomes an opportunity—to boldly push the refresh button and reinvent ourselves. My suggestion, no matter how close you are to actually retiring and what your state of mind, is to "retire from retirement."

"Retiring from retirement" means rejecting the cultural prescription for what you're *supposed* to do and doing what you want to the extent that is possible. Let's take a good hard look at your driving motivation—and your budget. If money is not a factor, do you feel that you have to keep working in order to maintain a sense of identity and busyness even though you'd actually like to retire? Or do you feel that you *have* to retire when you really don't want to, because you're "too old" to keep working? It's time to chuck that notion, too.

The traditional retirement age of sixty-five was set in 1935 when Social Security was born. Then we went ahead and built our whole society around the expectation that we'd be old and burned out by our mid-sixties. In 2016, though, the concept is a tad outdated. (Just ask Natasha.) Happily, this chapter (and this book) is about replacing our broad cultural assumptions with a philosophy and a plan that's tailor-made for you. And that's what The New Old is all about.

Over the course of reading this book, you've been drafting and revising a personal vision for your future. The core wisdom behind this is that you know best. By creating your *own* road map, you have determined that neither an archaic yardstick of the Social Security Administration nor our cultural biases nor anything or anyone else should tell you what this next phase of your life should look like. Of course, life will have its say. But it's up to you to design your own future.

So whether you really want to keep working—and society has been telling you to do otherwise—or whether you want to get the heck out of the workforce but feel afraid to make that leap, it's time to step back from the hubbub and tune in to the way you feel. And what you really want.

Take the time now to picture your best possible future. Perhaps your professional life has played an outsized role in your sense of who you are. Or your self-worth really is so tied up in what you do, or did, for a living, it's hard to picture yourself being happy doing anything else. If you're more like the rest of us, and you've used your professional life or role as a parent as a primary source of identity and self-worth for decades, take this opportunity to begin exploring and tapping other rich sources of self-worth, health, and satisfaction: community, spirituality, and setting healthier boundaries with your family are just a few possibilities.

And as you begin to draw this more expansive view of the future, circle back to the notion of "retiring from retirement." Once you've begun to disentangle yourself from the work-as-identity trap, you can take a more clear-eyed look at what retiring from retirement means for you personally. Maybe to you it's an enormous relief to finally take your foot off the pedal and cast off the responsibilities of work; maybe what you want most of all at this stage is to travel, play tennis, and hang out with your family. Maybe doing your job is the way you truly enjoy spending your days, and you want to keep doing it for as long as you can. If that's the case, *mazel tov*! Or there might be another option— or notion—worthy of exploring that's sitting there just outside of the box, waiting until now for you to discover it. Even if it doesn't have a name, take a few moments to give this notion some consideration. And while we're at it, let's explore some other unconventional ways of freeing up energy for the years ahead.

VOICING THE OBJECTION

Audacious or not, we know that aging isn't just a happy stroll through the park. Aging brings a slew of challenges and hardships, many of which we've touched on in this book. Part of being irreverent and audacious is having the courage to voice our objection. And say our "Aw shucks."

After an intimate relationship that lasted practically as long as I've been alive, Natasha lost her husband, Herman. And no matter how vivacious Natasha is to this day, she will never be the same as she was before Herman died. "Damn!"

For her entire life, my friend Amy relied on her impeccable memory. It made her great at her job and ultra dependable. Now, suddenly, she can't remember things. She's afraid. And she's angry that it was part of her memory, of all things, that the universe took from her first. "Damn it!"

I've also seen many friends my age who are vibrant and full of life suddenly begin to grapple with the painful physical changes that accompany aging. For some, hiking with me is no longer an option. They had felt so strong and self-reliant—and then, all at once, that changes.

In these cases, and many others, we have to be able to voice our displeasure, exasperation, humiliation, and anguish, rather than stuff it. Give yourself permission to voice your objection to the losses, setbacks, hardships, and disappointments in your life, and do it in a way that clears the air, opening a path for newfound strength, sensitivity, awareness, humility, and courage. Sometimes we have to spit in the face of the universe and say it out loud when our circumstances are just plain awful. No rationalization, no justification, no spin, just the objection. Give yourself permission to say it, speak it, tell it, shout it out loud, "This sucks!"

Strange though it may seem, we've got to be able to voice our objection in this way—because it's the counterpoint to expressing gratitude. In both, we are honest about what we're facing, whether it causes us grief or joy. As we have pointed out before, that raw honesty that allows us to give voice to our deepest sadness in the worst times and grants us permission to express our outrage in a constructive manner also allows us to fully experience our gifts and blessings in the good times.

May the expression of self-compassion, kindness, irreverence, outrage, and audacity open a world of gratitude and joy to you.

Chapter 11

THE CHANGING LANDSCAPE OF OUR RELATIONSHIPS AS WE AGE: AGING PARENTS, PARTNERS, AND ADULT CHILDREN

If you don't have love in your life, no matter what else there is, it's not enough.

—Mother Theresa

I had just moved from New York to rural Colorado for graduate school when my wife and I were invited to a welcome dinner. On our way to the dinner in my 1968 mustard-yellow Volvo, I got us lost on a winding road. Finally, I pulled over to ask for directions.

The person I stopped to ask was an older man who was standing next to his pickup truck. "How do you get to Monte Vista?" I asked.

"It's up the road about eight Cs," he said, smiling. "Just past the Mobil station."

I was confused. What did he mean by eight *C*s? Trying not to sound too much like a helpless city slicker, I asked, "Sir, I'm not sure what you mean by a *C*."

Again he smiled, and then he patiently explained that a *see* is a stretch of road that you can see in front of you. When you get to the end of one see, there's another see, and so on.

Sure enough, our dinner destination was eight sees up the road.

The process of aging, along with the shifting ground in our relationships as we age, is like a succession of sees on the road. At any given moment, we see a stretch of life ahead of us, like the horizon as the sun rises and sets each day. That stretch of life looks quite different than the stretch we saw ten years ago, and it's different from the stretch we'll see a few years from now.

This chapter is about navigating our relationships as they change from one see to the next, and doing so with the goal of leaving something I call a "legacy of love." What we can be certain about is that the landscape of our lives will change; we will change, our loved ones will change, and our relationships to one another will certainly change. Our relationships lead us down a sacred path of humility and wholeness, integrity, and vulnerability.

This chapter will show you how to temper and nurture your relationships—and set the stage for leaving a legacy of love. This means caring for your relationships with forethought and compassion—so that when your time comes, to the greatest degree possible, you and those you care most deeply for are left with a deep and abiding sense of spiritual connection. Or, as my friend Terry used to say, "Isn't it love that pierces the veil separating life and death?"

LEAVING A LEGACY OF LOVE: HONORING OUR RELATIONSHIPS WITH AGING PARENTS AND ADULT CHILDREN

When my mother moved from the cold winters of New York to the warm winters of California, I became her primary caregiver. She moved into a retirement community that provided her with all the amenities she loved and where her West Coast children, grandchildren, and great grandchildren could see her often. I made a point of coming to visit her frequently, and it was a blessing to have my mom so close. But something that needed attention kept putting a dark cloud over our visits.

When it was time for me to leave, I'd say, "Mom, I have to go now," and her face would fall. And after every visit I'd climb into my car with a heavy heart, feeling like I hadn't done enough, or given her enough time. This weighed on me and I decided to have a conversation with her. During our next visit, I sat down with my mother and explained:

"Mom, every time I tell you I have to leave, I can see how sad and disappointed you are. And it makes me sad. So how about this: Every time I'm going to visit, I'll call you and tell you in advance how much time I have. I'll tell you, 'Mom, I have an hour and a half.' And if that's okay with you, I'll come as scheduled. If that's not okay, I'll wait and come on a day when I have more time. I'll tell you, 'Mom, today I have *two* and a half hours. Is that OK?' "

She listened to what I said, nodded, and told me that we had an agreement. When I called in advance of a visit, she almost always said, "Great! An hour and a half will be wonderful." Sometimes, when the end of our visit rolled around, she'd play a little game to get me to stay later—suggesting that we have a meal together, or that I go say hello to her latest new friend—but when I reminded her of our agreement, she always nodded.

"We made an agreement," she would say. "That's fair."

And though our situation wasn't perfect, that simple act of making an agreement turned a difficult and heart-heavy circumstance into a much happier one. Mom and I could enjoy our time together, and though each of us always felt a tinge of sadness when I had to leave, it was also sweet.

That was not the only agreement that my mom and I made in the last years of her life. Even before she moved into a retirement home, my once brash and confident mother had started to wonder if she was becoming a bit inappropriate in certain social situations. We had talked on several occasions about how she was becoming increasingly "chatty," and even sometimes "unfiltered" in what she chose to say. She would talk over other people, causing family to no longer automatically invite her to family gatherings or friends at the retirement village to no longer include her at the dinner table. My once universally liked social butterfly of a mother began to feel lonely. It was very hard for her to admit it to me, but she eventually acknowledged that she was spending more time alone and feeling very down.

We made a plan together. After a few practice sessions, including some resounding belly laughs about her refurbished listening skills, my mother boldly set out to become more sociable. She focused on being a better listener, and I pledged to provide her with "reality checks" when we were out together; that is, I half-jokingly promised to tell her if she was "behaving" and that I would be checking for "scar tissue" on her tongue to make sure she was biting it.

It worked. My mother began listening more and watching her words. The results were immediate. She started getting more invitations, felt more included and, not surprisingly, her spirits lifted. "How did I do tonight, Zees?" (her affectionate nickname for me) she'd ask, smiling over at me after a family gathering.

"You were wonderful, Mom," I would tell her on most (but not all!) occasions. "Just wonderful?" she would joke.

We all need trusted confidants over the course of a lifetime. But there's a special place in heaven for trusted confidants who provide us with reality checks as we age. You see, we often lose our "filters" as we get older and can become more uninhibitedly direct, irritable, brash, and even crude. Who is going to tell us if/when we are going over the line, are talking too loud or have told the same story ten times? Who will tell us when we're being impossible or unreasonable? Or when we didn't accurately hear what was said and went off on a tangent, or began talking about another subject entirely? Everyone needs reality checks, especially in our later years, and I was honored to be able to provide that in loving tones for my mother.

As my mom continued to age, however, a very different kind of problem presented itself.

I was at a festive holiday party a number of years back when my cell phone (set on "stun") started vibrating. It was Janelle, the head of independent living at my mother's retirement community.

"Hi, Ken, I'm sitting here with your mom," she said, "and she's been in the lobby waiting for you to pick her up. She's worried something must have happened to you and seems a little confused. We're trying to reassure her that you're okay and to go back to her apartment, but I thought you might like to speak with her." With that, she put my mother on the line.

"Hey, Mom," I said in my most calming voice. "I wanted to tell you that I'm okay. What's going on?"

My mother's voice was trembling in a way that I had never heard. "Where are you?" she asked. "You were supposed to pick me up!"

We had no such plan, of course. I sensed that my mother had become very disoriented, and my heart sank into my stomach.

"I'll be right there, Mom. I'm coming to be with you. Go back to your room and I'll be there as soon as I can." I left the party, jumped in my car, and sped south.

My mother had always been sharp as a tack. I had never known anything but her keen sense of where she was, what time it was, and what was going on around her. This sad and unsettling episode at the holiday party turned out to be the first of several episodes in which my mom became disoriented. Each time, I would feel the sadness of a son whose parent was slipping away. And I would also feel the unspeakable joy when she would seem to come out of it and be her old ornery self.

The painfully uncomfortable question that most adult children of aging parents ask themselves at times like this is, "What, if anything, can I do?" There are no perfect answers, of course. Neurological examinations, testing, and trips to our family doctor confirmed that at ninety-two years old, my mom had some "slippage" in her cognitive functioning (much like my friend Amy). Our disheartened family simply did its best as each episode arose, reassuring my mother to soften the discomfort and disorientation she must have felt. There were times when no one could get there to be with her and times, like the holiday party, when I or someone else rushed over and held her hand.

I've learned that, as your aging parent is debilitated, experiences dementia and/or moves closer to the end of life, everything begins to flash before you: What you didn't do. What you wish you, and they, had done differently. For me the thing that became most salient in my reflections was a feeling that I had been too hard on my mom at times. I was too quick to fault her when I could have been more loving and patient.

Talking about this with others in the "Raising an Aging Parent" workshop I would offer residents and their families at my mom's retirement community, I discovered that this is a common sentiment; we all have our regrets. Things we'd like to do over. I used this new awareness to guide me in my last months with my mom. Being more patient and loving whenever we were together was my legacy of love to her. And the way she spoiled me, and showed me her affection and appreciation in our times together, was part of *her* legacy.

When my mom passed away last year, we celebrated her life, reviewing all of its chapters, from playing clarinet in the 1934 World's Fair to starting winter coat drives for the homeless wherever she lived. Grateful for the incredible generosity she showed our family, blessed by the depth and breadth of her intelligence and personality, and stunned by the reality that she would only be with us in spirit from then on, our family has laughed and cried a lot this past year. Above all else, I miss the twinkle in her eyes and smile when we'd share that special kind of love that exists between a mother and a son at any age. Right next to a picture I have on my desk of my daughters, I have one of my mother and me sharing exactly that kind of moment.

I've always kept pictures and mementoes from different parts of my past. In an old suitcase are old letters, the Torah from my bar mitzvah, trophies and medals, certificates of graduation and other pieces of my life through which I have constructed my sense of who I am. I've kept these things to help me remember, cherish, and review the years and seasons of my life. Add to them the photos, wall hangings, and artwork I have hanging on the walls of my home on my desk and in safe storage.

Now, as I get older and inherit treasured items of my parents', grandparents', and yes, my daughter Jenna's lives, I'm no longer just hanging on to my own archives. There is even a small wooden box of beautiful blond hair I found of my mother's, from when she was twenty, and slightly graying hair from when she was forty, and gray hair from when she turned eighty. Finally, she had a lock of beautiful gray hair from when she reached ninety. Strange as it may sound, I keep all these clips of hair my mother had saved in a box to track her journey through life in my safe.

On the one hand, I gladly and proudly accepted the mantle of maintaining our family archives. On the other hand, my garage, closets, and shed are now bulging with an astonishing amount of *stuff*. And if I don't do anything to organize it all, then I'll pass an impossible burden on to my fiancé, surviving daughter, and nephew, who in all likelihood will be the ones to clean out my house when I'm gone.

Putting my house in order, as we have discussed throughout these chapters, is my responsibility. As we've talked about in previous chapters, and as we'll get into in more detail in Chapter 13, each of us has a responsibility to take good care of our corner of the world for the next generation, and for the all the generations to follow. And this extends all the way to how I will organize and unclutter my house and go through my stuff.

I've actually hired someone to come in and help me organize and declutter, to get rid of things that aren't really important. To purge files. To organize and digitize what's left to create a functional, accessible family archive that can be enjoyed and passed on with love. This has become a priority.

TALKING AND LISTENING: OPENING THE LINES OF COMMUNICATION WITH LOVED ONES

Decluttering isn't only about our possessions. We can become a burden on others, and not just when it comes to inheriting the job of going through our stuff. Let's explore some of the other ways we want to avoid becoming a burden to our children as we age, beginning with being non-communicative about important things that really need to be discussed.

We may relish our independence, our resourcefulness, and our self-sufficiency. But our bodies and minds will change as we age just as they did for our parents and their parents. The key to staying ahead of the pain curve is to communicate in a timely and caring manner. Maintaining open and honest relationships with our adult children, and talking about the future, are best practices for preventing us from avoidable conflicts and impasses—and from becoming a burden on them! Besides being like the son I never had, my son-in-law, Tony, is a very successful estate planning attorney in La Jolla, California. Tony asks his clients to discuss a host of questions (he calls them "hypotheticals") with their families as an essential part of the planning process. Since some families and/or their situations do not lend themselves to open discussion, Tony masterfully facilitates conversations about touchy subjects with his clients privately, or, when possible, in family council meetings, where they become safe, productive, and open-ended discussions between family members.

Communication around important issues like the ones Tony and I came up with, listed below, is critical to effective estate planning. To best insure that you leave a legacy of love rather than one of loose ends, take time out with your family to talk about these things. Ask your estate planning attorney and/or a family specialist to help facilitate these discussions if necessary. Avoid the treachery that befalls too many conflict-avoidant families (and companies) by opening discussion on the hypotheticals. On the following pages is a sampling of conversation openers taken from our booklet *Psychological Estate Planning* (a subject I deal with extensively in the next chapter), to get you started:

Conversation Openers

1. I'm considering leaving you something as an inheritance. How do you feel about sitting down and talking about this?

2. What would you consider to be a fair and equitable distribution of our family wealth, both now while I'm here and after I am gone?

3. Is there anything of mine that you'd like to have after I'm gone? Please tell me what it is and why it's important to you.

4. Please tell me what you think I want for each of you, and our family, when I'm no longer here.

5. How do you feel about some of our family wealth being left to charities that I believe in?

6. Can I trust you to carry out my wishes after I'm gone? Or is there something that might stand in the way of doing that?

7. What might stand in the way of, sabotage, undermine, or turn my "Legacy of Love" estate plan into a nightmare for our family?

8. What, if anything, can we do now to insure that will not happen?

9. What steps would each of you be willing to take to make sure my wishes for our family are fulfilled?

10. Do you understand my good intentions—and the steps I've taken to make sure things work out for the best when I'm gone?

• • • • •

These are just a sampling of questions that foster open discussion, analysis, exploration, risk analysis, decision-making, and midcourse corrections. They are a perfect complement to more technical, legal, and financial stipulations; position statements; decisions; and desires you wish to share.

As with everything unforeseen, challenges and conflicts can arise. Perhaps one of your kids gets into trouble, showing themselves to be untrustworthy. Or the family business goes through a period of unexpected decline, forcing you to scrap or modify your succession plan. Having lines of communication open and clear agreements in place with your family members can play a vital role in keeping your family together—just the way they did with my mother.

And then there's the matter of communicating your innermost needs and wishes while you are alive. On your side of the ledger, perhaps you'd like more time with your grandchildren, or to make sure your adult children continue to treat you with respect as you get older. Maybe you want to make sure that you never become a burden to your spouse or kids. And then there's the matter of their needs and wishes. They might want to clarify their desire to take care of you as you get older or to redirect the family business after you have stepped back.

The work that you've already done to get your financial, legal, and medical house in order, back in Chapter 9, and open the lines of communication has given you a good start. But part of your legacy of love is communicating with your children about the ordinary business of life: What you each need, how you each want to be treated, and how you'll care for one another as things continue to change.

NAVIGATING OUR CHANGING RELATIONSHIPS WITH ROMANTIC/LIFE PARTNERS

Devastated by her husband Steve's Alzheimer's disease, a woman by the name of Lisa sought my help.

"Our marriage was a forty-year love affair," she told me as she described their relationship. "We could not be more adoring of one another."

At 6'4", Steve was a powerhouse of man whom Lisa had always looked to for strength and support. Now she was forced to watch the love of her life slip away, and she was devastated. The future they had planned together would have to be abandoned. The intimacy that was woven into the fabric of their every day was disappearing.

Then came a surprising moment. They were tearfully gazing at one another on the way home from a doctor's appointment. And that was when Lisa saw and felt something different than she ever had before.

"That look," Lisa told me, "meant everything. I know in that look that Steve will be with me forever."

Their relationship could never return to what it had been. Yet in the face of that loss, Lisa found the greatest peace and comfort that she could.

A host of issues arise when one partner falls sick. A debilitating disease may thrust one partner in the role of caregiver while the other partner succumbs to circumstances beyond his or her control. In addition to a sense of loss and heartbreak, the caregiving partner may also begin to feel a sense of resentment and betrayal: *This is not what I signed up for.* We aren't ready to relinquish our normal lives—and yet this is what we must now do. We may do our best but we don't like it one bit. In our moment of utter helplessness, and feeling powerless to save someone we love, we have every right to object. "Damn!"

Just as there were no perfect answers to the question of how to help my mom in her painful moments of disorientation, there are, of course, no simple answers as we watch a beloved partner struggle with illness—and as we're called to give up a part of our own lives, and our dreams, in the process.

These kinds of "living losses" are even more common in "age-different" relationships where there's at least a ten-year age gap between partners. I'm older than my fiancé, Lisette, and while I'm thrilled at the prospect of our future, I dread ever becoming a burden on her as we get older.

Both because of our age difference and the difference in life expectancy for men and women, it's overwhelmingly likely that she'll end up taking care of me towards the end of my life. That possibility scares me. Instead of secretly carrying that fear around with me and feeling embarrassed, I took a chance and confessed it to Lisette. In fact, we both wrote out our fears about aging, and then we sat down and shared our thoughts with each other. This was a huge step forward for us. Not only did it give us both a chance to voice our fears, we openly discussed things like these:

What if you or I get sick?
What if you or I get dementia?
What if one of us is debilitated by a stroke or a heart attack?
What if one of us gets cancer, or some other debilitating disease, like my friend Sam?
And of course: What if I die?

Once we'd both written our fears out and talked, we were able to say how we felt and what we wanted. Of course it wasn't news to her that she might end up in the caretaker role. And she reassured me that she would take care of me—just as I told her I would take care of her if she were to become ill or in any way debilitated.

We also talked about what had happened to my friend Sam after prostate surgery in his late seventies. Sam had described the depth of love he felt towards his wife and how spooning and caressing one another at night gave them an even deeper sense of connection and pleasure than sex. I shared the wisdom that Sam had imparted to me with Lisette: that some of life's greatest opportunities for true love and intimacy come when we're most vulnerable.

After having those conversations, my worry meter dropped from an eight all the way down to a three. Lisette will likely end up taking care of me, but who knows in this crazy life. I no longer fear becoming a burden to her, and, after a recent health scare, Lisette knows "in sickness and health" I have the capability and am committed to taking care of her should the need arise. Being open about all this has allowed us to turn our focus to the gratitude we feel right here, right now, instead of dwelling on the misfortunes of a hypothetical future.

In the next chapter we'll talk in greater detail about expressing love and gratitude to the important people in our lives now—and making amends wherever necessary.

SHIFTING
GEARS

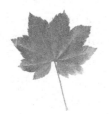

Chapter 12

PACK YOUR BAGS, THEN GO HAVE FUN: PSYCHO-SPIRITUAL ESTATE PLANNING

It's not enough to have lived. You have to have served others.
—Nelson Mandela

M y friend Walter Green was in his mid-seventies when he decided to pay homage to every person who had been a major influence in his life. After making that decision, Walter then actually visited *every last person* who he felt had earned that status in his life. He went around the world, visiting one special person at a time and telling them how much they'd meant to him.

Then he wrote a heartfelt book about the experience called *This is the Moment! How One Man's Yearlong Journey Captured the Power of Extraordinary Gratitude.* The first chapter is titled "An Idea Whose Time Has Come," and I couldn't agree more with that sentiment. The time *has* come for this idea—for each of us to pay tribute to (and/or make amends with) those whom we've known, or loved, or who have helped us along the way.

This process is part of something I call *psychological estate planning*. Back in Chapter 9 we talked about putting your house in order in the sense of your *legal* estate plan and your finances as well as your medical affairs. Now we turn to estate planning in a deeper sense: the psychological and spiritual estate planning of making sure things are sitting right in your relationships and in your heart.

Make no mistake about it, the work we do on ourselves to be psychologically at peace and in harmony with our loved ones is a huge part of our house, and our legacy. As we accept that we won't be around forever, the importance of tending to unfinished business in our relationships and with ourselves becomes clearer all the time. Taking care of business now—so we can have fun and be at peace in the years to come—is a wise investment.

In the pages to come we'll explore the benefits of expressing gratitude to those who've been there for you, introduce several effective ways of doing it, including *writing the* letter to your family and show the power of apologizing, forgiving, letting go, ending wars, making amends, confessing the truth, and reconciling differences.

LEAVING A LEGACY OF LOVE: MAKING AMENDS

We'll start with the process of making amends with the people in your life that really matter but with whom you have had a rift. Then we'll turn to expressing love and gratitude akin to Walter's round-the-world journey.

Drawing up a list of people you care about but with whom you have unresolved issues might be one of the more difficult things you have ever been asked to do. Even if you think there's no possible resolution in your relationship with a particular person, include him or her on the list. It might even be someone who has passed away. I affectionately refer to this as my "sh** list" because I feel crappy (pun fully intended) when things go sideways in relationships with people I care about—and don't really know what it might take to resolve our differences. It may be upsetting just to put down their name because it brings you back to a time of hurt, trauma, humiliation, rejection, betrayal, rage, and/or embarrassment. Remember you're doing this to make amends and possibly even heal a few wounds. Do your best to lean into or breathe through the feelings that are being triggered and write down all the names anyway.

You may feel you owe some people on your list an apology. Or that they are the ones who owe you an apology for something unforgivable they said or did long ago. Perhaps you allowed something to build up over the years instead of clearing the air with a close friend or family member. Putting a wall between the two of you and holding a grudge against them has effectively pushed them out of your life.

Then, one at a time, think about what, if anything, might be said or done to put this behind you. To get you started, fill in the blank to the following questions:

"If only they would _____, I might be able to put this behind me."

"If only I _____, we might be able to put this behind us."

"It would take _____ for me to forgive them for what happened."

"It would take _____ for me to forgive myself for what happened."

You're not looking for perfection. You are looking for reconciliation and some measure of peace knowing you said and did what you needed to. And that they were able to do the same. This transformational process of reconciliation works best when there's been thoughtful deliberation before the statement of apology or forgiveness and when you have set a positive tone. No matter what the circumstances of your relationship with a person, your deliberation might begin with an important first step: stating your intention of bringing matters to a positive outcome. It's easy to jump into the fray of a historically conflicted relationship and get caught up in who was right or who was wrong. Instead of focusing on who's the good guy and who is the bad, try to remember that the underlying purpose of this work is to clear the air. Forging peace is your reason for making amends with each person on the list.

After you've taken the time to deliberate and set the right tone, you're ready to either begin approaching the people on your list or reconcile what happened in the privacy of your own heart. No matter which you decide on, listen to the voice in you that seeks peace and understanding, not the one that harbors anger, resentment, vengeance, or fear. When you've decided what you want to say and how you want to say it, temper your words and tone by staying open and humble, inviting and forgiving, interested and accessible. Doing so disarms former adversaries and heightens the possibilities for understanding, forgiveness, reconciliation, and peace.

If you're going to make an apology to restore your integrity and revive a once-special friendship, for example, you might begin by saying, "I owe you an apology. I haven't been brave or confident enough to bring something up with you, and as a result, it has put a wedge in our relationship. I'm here because

I don't want anything standing in the way of our friendship anymore."

Perhaps you're apologizing for being judgmental. You might say, "When you and your wife split, I judged you and took her side. I'm ashamed and embarrassed that I did that. I want to tell you how sorry I am. And I'm hoping to make it up to you by promising that I'll never allow judgment to come between us again." What comes through most clearly is your tone when conveying how much this person means to you and how remorseful you are for what you did.

Many years ago, I had to make such an apology to my daughters. During a time when my marriage was struggling, and to compensate for the absence of connection I felt with my wife, I had unknowingly placed a weight on my daughters; I had invested all of myself and my energy into the lives of my children, because they were my greatest source of joy. And while this came from a place of love, it put an unfair burden on the two of them. This was a very difficult conversation to have, as I'm sure you can imagine. But after I spoke truthfully about what had happened and they had their say about what had happened, my girls expressed a deep sense of appreciation for what I had done to take ownership and responsibility for that painful part of our family's past. Part, if not all of the burden had been lifted, and I felt back in integrity with my girls. And indirectly with my ex-wife.

When there have been years of conflict or hard feelings, the first conversation may not get it all done. It may only be a humble beginning: an opening. And that's entirely okay. Say how you hope your message will be received and state your desired positive outcome. In my case it was, "I don't want anything standing in the way of our relationships, now or ever. And that's why I wanted to have this talk."

In cases where you can't imagine opening a conversation with this person because of hurt that is so deeply rooted in the past, you may want to consider bringing in a mediator. The presence of a neutral third party can help bring an otherwise impossible conversation into the light. A skilled mediator, facilitator, or family consultant must have the skill of a neurosurgeon in masterfully creating a safe atmosphere for all parties to say their piece and to be heard. Bringing intractable conflicts, differences, impasses, and wounds to resolution is considered by many a lost art; however, there are still talented attorneys like my son-in-law, Tony, and mediator/consultants, like yours truly, in your neck of the woods who can help your family.

How do you know whether you need a mediator? Think about whether it's reasonable to expect that you can work things out on your own. Then get a second opinion from someone you trust, perhaps even a level-headed family member or advisor. If it sounds to them like a mediator is a good idea, and you agree after having thought it through, give it a whirl.

With or without a mediator, though, this is a very delicate process. It includes not just apologizing but also offering forgiveness to those who may have wronged you in the past. Sometimes that feels all but impossible. The hurt and conflict are irreconcilable, the transgressions unforgivable. And such a meeting might actually be counterproductive. Some of us will have to make do, and find peace, in our own hearts, while others will be fortunate enough to discover that the solution was only a humble, sincere "I'm so sorry" away.

If you're not sure that you *can* forgive someone, start by asking what's at stake for you. Ask yourself, "What's at risk if I forgive this person? What's at risk if I *don't*?" Often, the thing that's at stake when we forgive someone is something that we've held on to for a very long time: a feeling of resentment, or that we were right and they were wrong. On the other hand, if we don't forgive, what's at stake is our relationship with that person and the possibility of having an unencumbered friendship with them once again.

It might seem counterintuitive, but the best reason to forgive someone is to give a gift to yourself. There's an old saying: "Forgiveness frees the forgiver." That's profoundly true. Finding the generosity to forgive will most of all serve you, because you will no longer carry that heavy burden around inside of you. You will have found the bigness of heart to let go of the anger you have harbored for those who have hurt, betrayed, or treated you poorly, and you will feel lighter for it. When it comes to family, finding forgiveness is part of the legacy of love. So much good can come simply from acknowledging and valiantly attempting to heal a family feud or neutralize long-standing family jealousies.

You might also find that just naming the elephant in the room—the conflict that's gone unspoken for so long—defuses much of its power. When you initiate a positive move such as asking for, or offering, forgiveness, that alone may take a lot of the oxygen out of the previous dark cloud of conflict. You may find that, even if things aren't perfect, they're much clearer and brighter than they've been in a long time. And that brings a much-needed lightness to your heart.

EXPRESSING LOVE AND GRATITUDE

What my buddy Walter did was extraordinary. I have since wondered: Why don't *all* of us do that? Why isn't it a rite of passage for each of us—like filing for Social Security?

It may not be realistic for many of us to spend a year seeking out and thanking every living person who played an important role in some stage of our lives. A simpler—and yet profoundly meaningful way of expressing gratitude and leaving your legacy of love is to write a letter that will stand as historical documentation of who you are, on whose shoulders you are standing, who and what you're grateful for, and what matters most. This document is the bible of your psychological estate plan: a clear and loving statement of what you choose to leave behind for the people who know and love you. And whom you adore.

So take some time, as we come to the end of this chapter, to jot down some talking points for what you might want your letter to say. If you're feeling bold and energized by the thought of doing this, consider writing a first draft.

There are beautiful examples of such letters written by those who have courageously faced the uncertain future. But the letter that stands in my mind as the most poignant example of a conscientious legacy of love was written by a twenty-year-old. And that twenty-year-old was my daughter Jenna.

The letter, which was addressed to "everyone in our family," is a lasting reminder of Jenna's love and what really matters in this life. Here is what my amazing daughter wrote two short weeks before she died:

> I am in South Africa right now, and I have just had the most incredible day of my whole life, and I feel so complete and so part of the world around me. I have visited such incredible places, it's almost unreal. Not incredible like Hawaii or Cancun or Europe, but places that make me feel human and connected to what is happening around me. And as I encounter these feelings, and people, and cultures I cannot help but reflect on my own background and my own roots.

I want my *whole* family to know how much I love all of you and how proud I am to be a part of this family. I know that I am crossing that road in my life where I am no longer a child and I am going to soon be going out into the "real world" where time is fast and busy (even more so than now). But I want you all to know how much a part of my heart you are.

I take you with me in all of my travels, journeys, and discoveries. I see such a pride in family in these other cultures I have visited and even though these people have nothing in terms of monetary objects, they have the priceless value of pride and strength in their family and their backgrounds. So as I visit with these people, I have reaffirmed my own path in what is real, who I am, and where I came from—and this is all of you.

My family is the greatest love I know and I will always be tied to it. I love you all and miss you incredibly.

Always,

Jenna

Leaving a legacy of love means having the important conversations that forge understanding and peace, making amends, saying the things we need to say from a loving heart, and blessing the life we've lived.

It means that we have, above all, expressed the full measure of our love and gratitude, leaving behind only a feeling of peace.

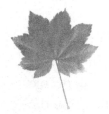

Chapter 13

SOCIAL RESPONSIBILITY: PAYING IT FORWARD

You can't live a perfect day without doing something for someone who will never be able to repay you.
—John Wooden

W hen I die, I want to go like my Uncle Fred, peacefully in my sleep. Unlike his passengers, who were screaming as the car went over the embankment."

I just love that joke. We have to be able to laugh about this stuff—and poke fun at life—or we'll go crazy!

In a funny way, the joke about Uncle Fred is also a great introduction to the conversation about social responsibility. Uncle Fred's final deed in this life is the antithesis of social responsibility, since he wasn't exactly giving back to those coming behind him!

The tidal wave of baby boomers now reaching retirement has been referred to as the "silver tsunami." With ten thousand

138

boomers turning sixty-five every day, and with many projected to live well past ninety, we're living in a time of great change. Government agencies are investing time and resources into answering the questions posed by this vast demographic shift, from health care to housing to financial management. You might even remember, back in Chapter 10, that I mentioned my friend Natasha (age ninety) is working with gerontologists at the University of California on the pressing issue of how cutting-edge technology can be harnessed to assist the elderly.

But as we ride this tidal wave into our latter years, the questions are not only about how society can and must change in order to accommodate these evolving demographics. The questions are also about what *we* must do to pay forward our assets and blessings (and hopefully they are abundant) to our heirs and to society. Indeed, we have an enormous collective responsibility.

We've spent a lot of this book focusing, in one way or another, on the expression of gratitude. In the last chapter you read about my friend Walter who went around the world thanking every person who had helped him, and then how you can draft your own letter of gratitude to your family. Well, now is the time to consider how you might channel your hard and soft assets, including your depth of experience, sage wisdom, special skills, newfound emotional freedom, and gratitude into making the world a better place.

Paying it forward—giving something back to the world that gave you life—is your ethical and moral, if not spiritual, responsibility. Taking steps to ensure the beauty in nature, majesty in the arts, divinity in human rights, and promise of an education being available to future generations is both an opportunity to go beyond yourself and be of service to others and your invitation to live with grace and nobility selflessly and philanthropically. Without expecting anything in return.

You have seen how offering forgiveness to someone who has wronged you is as great a gift to you as it is to the other person. A win-win proposition, if you will. So is fulfilling your social responsibility. At the same time you give something of value to a world that needs it and are profoundly nourished in the process. It's a heck of a deal.

FINDING YOUR SERVICE

I shared earlier how my mother's end-of-life decline happened only last year after a difficult period in which her always-sharp mind grew shaky and disoriented. What you don't know is that my mother was always my first and best role model for what social responsibility, or prosocial behavior, looks like.

My mom was ninety-two when she died. She spent seventy of those years bringing people of different religions and races together in our community. And fighting for social justice. When I was growing up in New York, my mother's volunteer work was a fixture in our household. Though there was a time when I was very young and didn't understand why this work took her away from our home, I soon learned. Having been brought up in the crowded back room of her parents' market, my mom had a deep and abiding appreciation for the simple things of life. Like her father, Jacob, whose brother Kaseal (for whom I'm named) died in the Holocaust, she was a true champion of the oppressed and disadvantaged. My mom was a bridge builder between people from different backgrounds. The importance of personal dignity, equality, and civil rights never eluded my mother. Right up to the end she was speaking out about how "our world is broken" and how "we need a new generation of visionary leaders to repair the hatred and violence."

My mom's dedication to the betterment of society as a bridge builder is one kind of service. Natasha's dedication to building bridges between generations is a whole other kind of service. Both represent a deep commitment to leaving this world better than they found it. And there are so many other worthy ways for us to give back; the type of service that's right for you will depend on what deeply moves you on a personal level, what you're capable of contributing, and the opportunities available for you to do so.

Consider, for instance, my friend Malin, who is eighty-eight—and a very generous man and visionary leader in our community. Malin made a lot of money in his career, but that's not what keeps him happy. Or busy. These days he's remarkably clear about what gives his life purpose.

"'Making our community a stronger, better, fairer version of itself over the years has given my life meaning," he told me recently. "Much more so than more money ever could have."

Malin's success in real estate afforded him the financial wherewithal to donate widely and generously to research institutions, schools, universities, and charities. He has helped to found several philanthropic organizations and is largely responsible for some of the best, most innovative entities in "America's Finest City." But this isn't a guy who gives a million dollars and then asks for his name to be emblazoned on the side of a building. He knows that's not what it's about. Malin humbly offers his financial resources and his management expertise to worthy organizations and their boards of directors because he knows he's contributing to something bigger than himself.

"I didn't want to make my work my life," he told me—which is quite a statement coming from a guy who was so successful. "I had other callings, and I wanted to leave enough time to pursue them.

I was blessed with abundance. And now I'm at peace knowing that I gave back."

Whether it involves feeding the homeless once a year on Thanksgiving, founding a Center for Civic Engagement (as Malin did), volunteering to adopt a family ravaged by terrorism, or donating time to the League of Women Voters, social responsibility is an important dimension of psychological estate planning. Remember that estate planning is not really about us; it's about those who will go on after us. Your efforts to make the world a better place before you depart are an integral part of your psychological and spiritual estate. How have you used your life to better others, and can you now rest easily in mind, body, and spirit?

So take some time to think about what your particular brand of service might look like. Perhaps you see yourself helping families in your community who are in need. Perhaps you have expertise like Malin's, and your contribution will be to sit on a board of directors and help steer a mission-driven organization. Maybe you want to swing a hammer and help build houses for Habitat for Humanity. Maybe you've wanted to get involved in disaster relief to help victims of a recent flood or hurricane, and you decide to coordinate a food and clothing drive. Or maybe you're part of a religious community, and you've always wanted to make time for the community service trips that your house of worship already organizes. You may have adopted or rescued a dog or cat from an animal shelter and wish to support their efforts. Or you set some time aside to help a program for foster kids trying to get into college.

Perhaps your service will be given to your own family as a grandparent, helping out as needed with grandchildren or fixing a few things up at your son or daughter's new house. Or maybe, given the state of the world, you will devote your time and energy to advocating for/working to protect civil and women's rights where you live. Whichever type of service you embrace, you'll find the world ready and grateful to receive your efforts.

If community service has always seemed somewhat onerous to you—like something you *have* to do instead of something you *want* to do—then take some time to cast a wide net. Nine times out of ten, you can find a way of volunteering that directly connects to something you're passionate about. Maybe it's helping out in the oncology unit at the children's hospital or mentoring kids in an art program at a local youth-serving organization. Maybe you're passionate about civic engagement, and you end up volunteering at your local polling place. Or your deep appreciation for, and love of, the arts inspires you to make sure they are taught in the schools where you live. Whatever it is, there's a way to be of service to the world *and* to follow your particular passion. And you'll actually be of greater service to the world this way—because you'll be far more effective at something you actually enjoy!

At its core, the ethic of social responsibility boils down to three fundamental ideas:

1. **We each have the ability to use our knowledge, skills, resources, and lifetime of experience to benefit others.**
2. **We choose not to lose sight of those who have less than us, and we become their stewards and advocates.**
3. **We have the power to make the world we live in more of what we want it to be by using our voices, standing up for what we believe in, and, to quote Gandhi, "Being the change we want in the world."**

BRINGING IT HOME

I've found that putting this ethic of social responsibility into action eventually starts to influence every other part of our lives. When we spend time helping others and give selflessly of ourselves, it naturally begins to spill over into our other activities, relationships, and world view.

Back in Chapter 11, I mentioned that I've essentially become my family's archivist. I have pictures of my grandparents and great-grandparents in Austria and Russia, coming through Ellis Island, all of which came into my possession after Mom passed away. I am also the keeper of my late daughter's legacy: housing everything precious that I could possibly keep from her life and storing the archives of The Jenna Druck Center for the past twenty years. But with countless crates and boxes of archives accumulating in my shed, garage, and closets, I could very easily end up inadvertently putting a great burden on my family.

This situation brings to mind two stories that might be cautionary tales for all of us.

Sadly, a colleague's wife, Carole, passed away last year. When sitting shiva (paying respect and mourning) at their home, my colleague half-jokingly told us she had been a pack rat and the kids had already begun uncluttering their home. "We're giving things to The Salvation Army and the rest is trash," he joked, adding, "This is definitely going to be a three-dumpster job!"

The second story involves the deathbed confession of an eighty-year-old man named Richard. Knowing the end was near, he sheepishly handed his daughter the key to a secret storage unit where he'd been hoarding things his wife assumed had gone to Goodwill all these years.

Are you a three-dumpster or secret storage unit person? I've concluded that I am, which is why I'm making a making a major effort to go through all my things, from files to clothes to old artifacts, and let go of things I no longer need. I've even hired a professional organizer to help me sort through and pare down all my stuff—and who is teaching me a lot about how to let go.

Whether it's physical clutter, or the kind we store from unresolved wounds and conflicts that we discussed in the last chapter, now is the perfect time for some much-needed spring cleaning and for upgrading our "letting go of stuff" software.

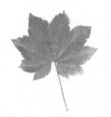

Chapter 14

FACING INTO THE INFINITE:
THE IMPERMANENT LIGHT
BURNING ETERNAL

Have patience with everything that remains unsolved in your heart . . . live in the question.
—Rainer Maria Rilke

About three weeks ago, walking past a mirror that I've passed a thousand times before, I saw something new. I had lost quite a bit of weight, and my face looked different. Thinner for sure. Although I received compliments like "You look so much younger," when I caught a glimpse of myself in the mirror, I looked a little gaunt. And that immediately triggered a memory of my father. In his last couple years of life, my Dad was struggling with congestive heart failure, looking gaunt and old.

It wasn't that I looked sick, staring back at myself in the mirror. But I did look a lot like my father as an older man. My dad was a big guy, over six feet tall and stocky (like I was, until recently).

But in his later years as his heart weakened, he began losing that extra weight. His smile had that radiant, ageless glow, but his face aged significantly.

I've come to the place in my life where I have begun to look like an older guy, and I see my father in me. This isn't a bad thing; catching a glimpse of my older self in the mirror, it's more eye-opening than unsettling or disturbing. Seeing the man I have become made me smile in a way that was eerily similar to my dad's. Witnessing this older version of myself melding with the older version of my dad, I saw that we belonged to something much bigger. I am Ken, the son of Charles. Charles was the son of his dad. And so on. My father and I, and the fathers before us belong to the ages. I had never felt connected to the expanse of life over the generations as I did in that moment, and ever since.

I saw in that mirror the big picture: that each of us is mortal, and yet we're also part of something bigger than us—something, ethereal, beyond perhaps our capacity to fully understand. Something mysterious, timeless and eternal. "And at the end of our lives," my friend Ken Blanchard reminds us, "Like all the pieces that come with Monopoly—the money, real estate, dice, and cards—it all goes back in the box." What matters most—that is never lost and never disappears—is the love.

We've come now to one of the most elusive parts of our psychological estate planning process: the spiritual part. We acknowledge that our lives are temporary, that life is a lease program and in the end, everything goes back in the box—except for love. Love never dies.

We also come to certain questions about who we have been during our time on earth. Have we, for example "been the best version of ourselves?" Are we proud of who we were as children to our parents, and as parents to our children? Were we good life partners, family members, friends and coworkers? Can we ultimately rest comfortably, knowing, as my dear friend Asa said to me at the end of his life, "We did good, Kenny!"

Delving into the spiritual nature of life, understanding and coming to terms with things we cannot know for certain, requires the ability and willingness to consider the paradoxical: Our existence here on earth is both impermanent and eternal. My daughter Jenna is both here and gone. My heart is broken, and yet it is more whole and full than ever before. Perhaps our ability to hold that paradox is a glimpse of the divine in each of us.

We spend a good part of this life learning to embrace our humanity and becoming the person we are. And then we get older. As we face into life's later seasons, we are asked to let it all go. This means surrendering who we've been all these years, including our identities, ego, and future plans. Making peace with death, the end of our physical existence as the man, husband, dad, brother, or friend—or the woman, wife, mother, sister, or friend—we have been. And embracing our place in the larger scheme of things, or, as some would say, our "beyond."

MAKING PEACE WITH OUR OWN IMPERMANANCE

For many of us, the issues in this chapter are inherently more difficult to wrap our minds and hearts around than others I have presented. You are a courageous person or you wouldn't have picked up this particular book (and you certainly wouldn't be so far into it). And yet it is part of our very humanity to fear the prospect of our own demise. Being steeped in a death-denying culture has only made our avoidance of and possible aversion to death even stronger. But I encourage you to keep pushing forward. Gently. The rewards of reducing or eliminating our fears around dying are many and worth the hard spiritual work it takes to get there. The benefits of being at peace—or having some measure of peace as we get older—can affect your quality of life in ways that cannot be underestimated.

In the following pages you will find a series of exercises. These exercises rest on the foundation of the considerable work you've already done to process what it is to be getting older. Now, though, we need to gently push ourselves even further, summoning the strength and the mental and spiritual toughness to squarely face and acknowledge our own mortality.

EXERCISES FOR FACING INTO OUR OWN IMPERMANENCE

Read through the following exercises, designed to open a line of inquiry, to see which ones resonate most with you, and then go from there.

1. **Embracing our aging bodies**

   Having watched our bodies change as we have gotten older (some of us have spent countless hours and energy obsessing about having a perfect body and beating ourselves up with harsh criticism), this is an opportunity to trade in the old way of seeing things. This new way allows us to see, forgive, accept, love, and cherish our older physical self and go beyond our fears.

   Complete the following sentences:

   - In the past I saw you as _____, and now I see you as _____.

   - In the past I have judged and rejected you for _____, and now I accept you as _____.

   - In the past I have denied _____, and now I embrace _____.

2. **Opening to our feelings of embarrassment and shame**

Our bodies tend to be one of our greatest sources of self-rejecting, self-loathing, shame, and embarrassment as we age. Consider the following:

- I might be embarrassed to admit it, but I still feel ashamed about _____.

- In order to no longer feel ashamed about this, I need to _____.

- One small step I could take toward doing this would be to ___

3. **Taking inventory of our true assets and worth**

The great wisdom of the Lakota Sioux spoken about earlier that "today is a good day to die" is a curious aspiration. When we dwell in gratitude, it becomes easier to see that today is complete and would, indeed, be a good day to die. Take a few moments now to take inventory of your assets, counting what *really* matters: the cherished people and things that have made life worthwhile. These blessings will all one day go back in the box because that is the way of life. And I will forever be grateful for them.

4. **Sitting with our uncomfortable feelings**

There are some parts of aging that we can learn to embrace, and there are other parts that we may never become entirely comfortable with. Perhaps it's a feeling of powerlessness or even helplessness as our bodies and minds change. Perhaps it's a lingering feeling of fear or dread. Some of us have long felt terrified by the prospect of growing old and dying. Go ahead and name the things you just can't seem to accept. Instead of trying to hide, deny, reject, or obliterate them, invite them in. Sit with them, allowing each one to surface in a way that awakens newfound awareness and bravery, invites a softening, and introduces an element of surrender. *Sitting with* is a bold and honest way for us to *be with* what is.

5. **Sharing and unburdening ourselves**

You don't have to do this alone! Identify a trusted partner, friend, or confidant with whom you can be entirely honest about your aging process. Ask for their ear and their counsel, and then unburden yourself of your lingering fears and discomforts. You can also get help dealing with fears about death from trusted clergy, professional coaches, and counselors who are master teachers. I personally have drawn great strength, courage, and perspective about death and dying from the sage wisdom of my dear friends John Welshons and Elisabeth Kubler-Ross as well as the humble teachings of Ram Dass and Stephen Levine.

6. **Accepting our elder status**

With a dose of humility and an even bigger dose of humor, see if you can embrace the idea of yourself as an elder. If that doesn't work, consider buying an "Old Fart" or "100 Percent Crone" T-shirt. Whether laughing at your wrinkles, staring down your old-seeming face in a shop window (I can relate!), giving yourself an audacious-sounding nickname or agreeing with your spouse to get tested for a hearing aid (which you've probably needed for years), it's time to lighten up and relax into being the older version of yourself. In addition to senior discounts, AARP perks, and getting the comfiest chair at family gatherings, there are some great benefits that go along with elderhood just waiting to be discovered when you're ready to tune into/harvest them. Just ask my friend Jim Selman, who founded The Eldering Institute, about the color and beauty of autumn leaves falling from the tree of life.

7. **Contemplating and reimagining our remaining years**
Using meditation, guided imagery, calming music, moments of silence, or something else that helps you cultivate stillness, quietly contemplate your remaining years. Allow yourself to imagine your best, worst, and probable future, one at a time. After each one, open your eyes and write down everything that happens in that future. Review the narratives for your best, worst, and probable futures and place your hand on your heart. Pray, hope, request, reimagine, or set your intention for your best possible future, exactly as you'd like it to go. And then breathe it in.

8. **Embracing our impermanence**
You've just captured some of your hopes and fears about what the future may hold. You've also logged what seems, from your present vantage point, to be your most likely path forward. Though we cannot know the future, we do know that we are all headed to the same place. Take some time now to sit with this non-negotiable reality, uncomfortable though it may be. If you find this kind of surrendering of control difficult, try to hold yourself extra close. And breathe. In your most gentle and reassuring voice, say something that softens your fears about this part of your passage through time. Perhaps something like "You're going the way of those you love who have gone before you. And you'll be followed by those who come after," "It's OK. This is the way of life," "Go with God," or Stephen Levine's assurance that "love is the bridge" will resonate with you and calm your heart. Search for the words

of reassurance and faith that bring you some measure of peace, like those of the great Persian poet, Rumi, who saw death as "our wedding with eternity." Rumi reminds us, "Goodbyes are only for those who love with their eyes. . . . For those who love with their heart and soul, there is no such thing as separation." Right next to your fear, hold the words that bring you some measure of comfort. Add to that the thoughts of how blessed you have been in this life. Imagine/see yourself at peace. At rest. And at ease. No longer having to suffer or struggle. Or fear the unknown. You have faith. Your heart is calm. And you are at peace.

9. **Being present and humble**

"Today is a good day to die" isn't only an invitation to embrace death—it's an invitation to live in the present as fully as we possibly can. So take a few deep breaths, and feel what it is to be alive at this moment. Feel the air moving effortlessly into and from your lungs and the relief of resting yourself on the chair beneath you. You have traversed the plight of our human existence, and, as my angel daughter's voice once reminded me, what you have ahead of you now is *more nows*. It's time to just allow yourself to be *here*. In the now. That's all there is, or ever was, so let it be.

• • • • •

In the next and final chapter, we'll look at strategies for cultivating your newfound peace, courage, gratitude, and wisdom in the moments, days, months, and years to come. Completing our soul's journey, making peace, and finding our way home are deeply personal matters that we're now ready to consider.

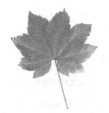

Chapter 15

COMPLETING YOUR SOUL'S JOURNEY: COMING HOME

When my time comes, there will be a hand reaching down for me, and it will be the hand of my daughter Jenna.
—Ken Druck

That a child I helped bring into this world died before me still breaks my heart. So does the thought of having to let go of my earth daughter Stefie's hand as I pass from this world. But the thought of Jenna's hand being there after I take my final breath gives me peace. The possibility of reuniting with my angel daughter after all these years bring me boundless joy and takes away my fear.

Can I be certain of that? No, and that's why we call it faith. As we come to the end of this book, and as we all contemplate the end of our own lives as we've know them, we arrive at the unfathomable part of the journey. Gazing at the infinite. The vast unknown. Or "the enormity" as Jenna calls it.

We belong to the ages. Beyond how we have come to know ourselves as individuals, we have a place in the great mystery of things. We may have already found peace and assurance in our faith. Or we may be coming to a time when we no longer feel so burdened by our unknowingness, or by our smallness in the universe, and we can make peace. At age sixty-seven, I am beginning to taste this kind of peace. I'm making peace with this life—and with the things I just don't know a damn thing about for certain. And that's OK.

And while this chapter is about completing your soul's journey, I am the first to admit that I don't know exactly what that completion looks like. It is easy to become attached to terms like *closure* and to imagine that there are certain right and wrong things to do as we come to the end of each season of life, and eventually the entire journey.

I choose to hold the notion of completion as a feeling—that we have done enough, and that we have come to where there is no visible "see" in the road ahead. No road map. No future plan. Not even the dim light of the stars to guide us. Only a faint hope that things turn out OK. We now allow ourselves to be at peace, knowing that we have done the best that we could. And that is enough.

FINAL QUESTIONS FOR MAKING PEACE

As we're poised here, contemplating the infinite, the following questions may help guide your thoughts:

- **Is there something beyond this life I can find peace in thinking about?**

- Can I find peace even without knowing for certain what will happen as I get older and eventually pass? If so, how can I cultivate it?
- If I had a month to live, what, if anything, would be weighing most heavily on my heart?
- What do I still need to do to make sure my "bags are packed?" What is the unfinished business of my life?
- Are there people I want to tell how much I love them or who I want to thank for loving me? If so, who are they and what do I need to say to them?
- Have I allowed myself to receive the full measure of love and gratitude that my family, friends, and others whose lives I've touched feel towards me? If not, what would it take for me to open my heart and finally let it in?
- Is there an essence about me, something bigger than my own life, that will live on? What words, symbols, or sounds would I use to describe it?
- Will I allow myself to entertain the possibility that there is nothing to fear about death, even if just for a microsecond (even if I am not certain about what death actually is)?

FINAL ACTIONS AND FOLLOW-UP

You were brave to pick up this book in the first place. Now you've maintained that courage through fifteen chapters and looked inward at some of the most difficult and vulnerable areas of life. I can only hope that you are feeling deeply proud of yourself for having made this literary pilgrimage.

Having a powerful experience is one thing. We've all been inspired by a TV show, movie, speech, or intimate conversation we've had with someone. And then, when we go back to our day-to-day lives, it slowly fades away. Follow-up is 75 percent of the battle. I make summary recordings of all my coaching sessions for my clients on voice memo so they will retain 50 percent more of what we said and did. In addition to keeping this book handy as a reference, here are three simple things that I am hoping will help you carry you forward and advance the growth you've made in this process of courageous aging:

- **Make an agreement with yourself to form what you've learned into newfound awareness, tools, and daily practices. Writing down concrete, specific steps for how you're going to prioritize and put into play what you have discovered is truly important.**

- **Hold yourself accountable for this plan to make the coming years of your life some of the best ever.**

- **Write a letter to your future self that details what you have committed to. Open the letter in six or twelve months and fine-tune the plan, making adjustments where necessary.**

- **Ask your spouse, friend, sponsor, confidant, or coach to support you in this grand adventure. Meet with someone who understands and can support your efforts on a regular basis. Solid support can make all the difference and help you remain accountable.**

- **Place your hand above your heart one more time and picture yourself feeling happy and at peace. Thank yourself for doing what's necessary to become the kinder, smarter, calmer, braver, and more loving version of who you are.**

- **Picture the smiling faces of all those people who love you and are deeply grateful to you. Allow yourself to feel their love. Let it in.**

HAPPILY NEVER AFTER

If you're like me, you love that *happily ever after* feeling at the end of a good book or movie. Everything is somehow going to work out and it's all going to be OK. And then we go back to real life.

In real life, we find peace and experience the fullness of life in one moment and find ourselves in a state of unrest, unknowingness, and even emptiness in the next. Being human is just that way. Life is just that way.

Following a path of courageous living and aging does not lead to *happily ever after*. There will be ups and downs, clarity and confusion, peace and unrest on the road ahead. Life will be life. And it is up to each of us to find some measure of peace in letting it be so.

MY PRAYER FOR YOU

My prayer for you is that you will unleash your potential for love, courage, clarity, and joy as you get older, and live each moment, day, month, and year as fully as possible. You will balance pushing yourself too hard (resulting in a yoga injury) with not pushing hard enough (because you're "too old" to take a yoga class). And if you're asked how old you are, you will now respond with a calm, knowing smile. With the completion of this last paragraph, I will hope to have done my very best to bring about an opening, a healing, a liberating, and a warm deepening in your life.

I wish you every happiness, every blessing and every measure of peace.

Ken Druck

PLEASE STAY IN TOUCH
www.kendruck.com
www.facebook.com/kendruck

If this book has been useful to you or someone you care about, please write and tell me. Not only do I want to hear from you, knowing that I've helped you become the better version of yourself will bring me great joy and satisfaction.

Please also share your stories and insights with me. And tell me about other valuable resources on this subject that you've discovered so I can share them with others.

If I can help you, your family, your business/organization, or community; speak/give a presentation for your group; tell you about Courageous Aging Workshops; or to start a Courageous Aging Discussion group in your community, please contact our offices at info@kendruck.com or by calling (858) 863-7825.

Thank you.

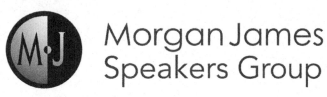

Morgan James
Speakers Group

www.TheMorganJamesSpeakersGroup.com

We connect Morgan James published authors with live and online events and audiences whom will benefit from their expertise.

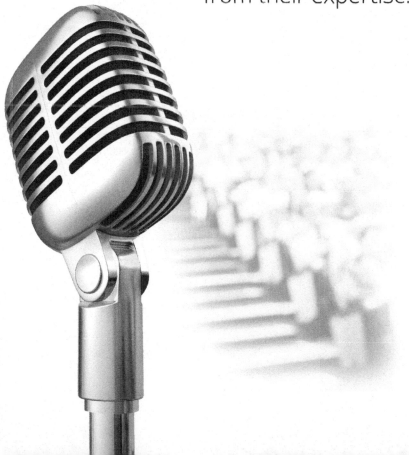

APR **1 9** 2019

CPSIA information can be obtained
at www.ICGtesting.com
Printed in the USA
BVOW08s1912221017
498349BV00002B/127/P